ESSENTIAL OILS FOR BEGINNERS

The Where To & How To Guide For Essential Oil Beginners

By Mary Jones

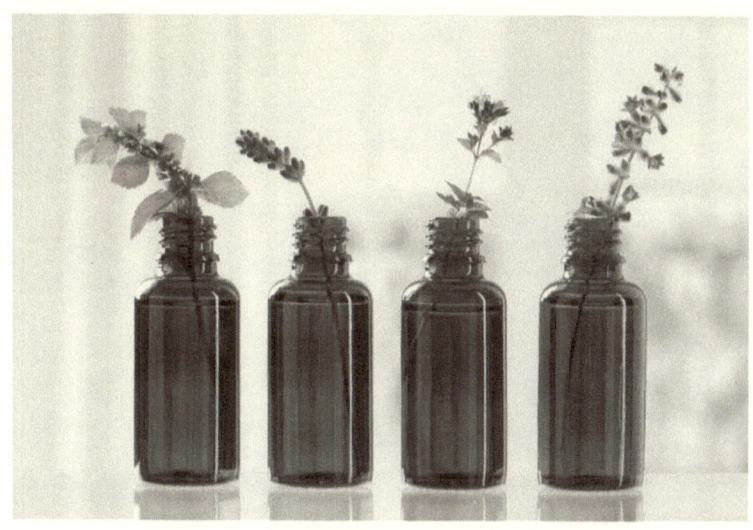

Essential oils have a bio-electrical frequency that is several times greater than the frequency of herbs, food, and even the human body. Clinical research has shown that essential oils can quickly raise the frequency of the human body, restoring it to its normal, healthy level.

TABLE OF CONTENTS

INTRODUCTION

In recent years, the amount of **people using alternative treatments** – including essential oils – for common ailments has increased dramatically (as shown by the example diagram below, *according to NCCIH at nccih.nih.gov, US, 2007*).

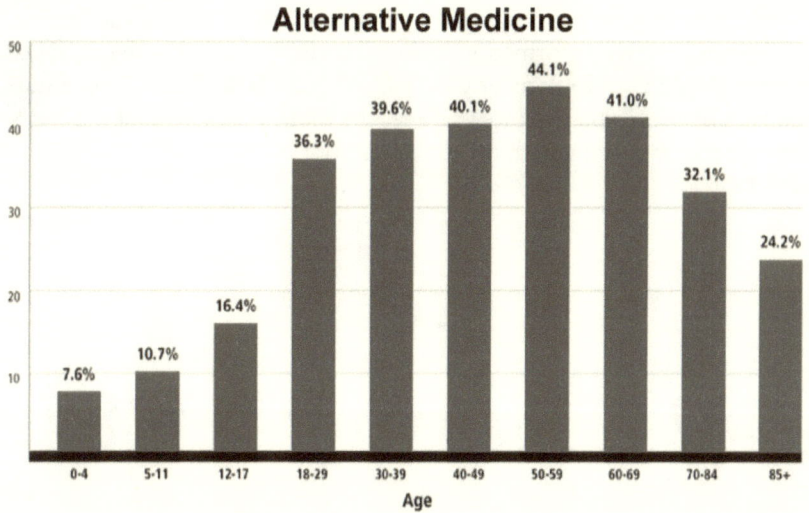

There are a number of reasons for this – which will be examined throughout the chapters of this book – but below are **the most common benefits** that people find **from making the switch to essential oils**. These include:

- ***Very Powerful*** – Essential oils can have a healing effect mentally, physically, and emotionally.

- ***Easy to Use*** – They can be used wherever you are, and the methods necessary to take the oils are very simple – wear them like perfume, use them in your home for cleaning or aromatherapy, or simply keep a bottle with you for inhalation or topical applications.

- *Highly Effective* – They can penetrate the skin and affect the emotional center. So they can help you handle stress, anger, or any other emotion.

- *Multipurpose* – You can make nontoxic, green household products by blending essential oils.

- *Heterogenetic* – Essential oils can have multiple properties, e.g. calming and grounding.

There are hundreds of thousands of uses for essential oils in health care, and these include stress relief, losing weight, and energy enhancement, just to name a few. This book will give you *all* of the information you'll need to get started using these oils – **what** to buy, **where** to buy them from, **recipes** for these common ailments, etc. – plus you'll be given a selection of **resources** to allow you to do some research of your own – after all, you aren't going to change your current healthcare plan without all of the necessary information!

You won't find a more comprehensive guide to essential oils on the market. Read through all of the information included in this book, and you might just find yourself willing to **look after yourself in a much healthier, more natural way**. The more you use essential oils, the more you'll see that the benefits work for your mood and mind, as well as your body. So, why not read on to learn more?

A QUICK GUIDE TO ESSENTIAL OILS

Essential oil is described as:

"An oil derived from a natural substance, usually either for its healing properties or as a perfume. Some pharmaceuticals, and many over-the-counter or 'holistic' remedies, are based on or contain essential oils. For example, products containing camphor or eucalyptus essential oils can help relieve congestive coughs, and many essential oils are used in the practice of aromatherapy."

Essential oils have been used for centuries for their healing and wonderful fragrant properties. There are literally thousands of ailments that can be helped with these essential oils, which will be examined in more detail throughout this book.

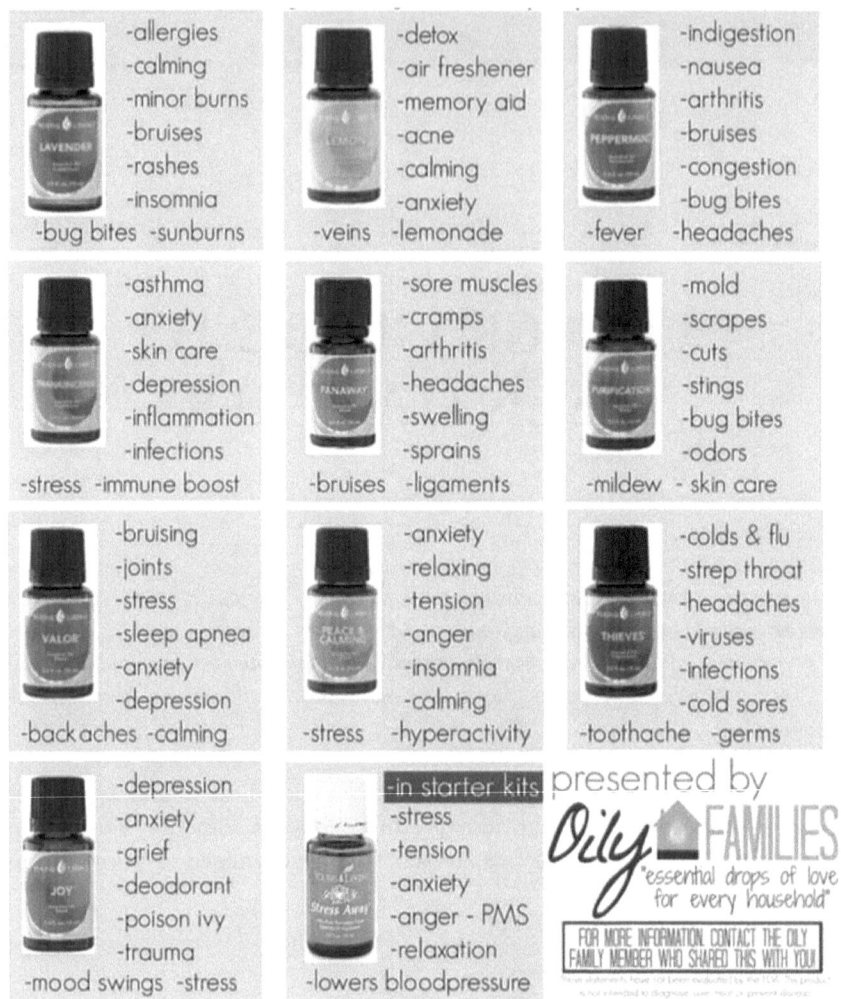

There is often a mix up with **'essential oils'** *and* **'aromatherapy.'** To clear that up right away, here is the definition of aromatherapy:

> *"**Aromatherapy** is a complementary therapy that involves the use of **essential oils**. It may be used to help improve both your physical and emotional well-being."*

Put simply, an essential oil is a natural plant compound, usually collected via distillation, that retains the distinct odor of the source plant it is extracted from.

What you might not know about essential oils is *they aren't actually oils!* They don't contain any of the fatty acids that constitute what we would consider an oil.

Essential, or volatile, oils are chemical-based liquids derived from plants that help create many smells we know and recognize. Essential oils are not considered "true" oils like Flaxseed or Olive oils, which are known as fixed oils. Fixed oils cannot vaporize like essential oils, because they are heavier. Volatile oils contain over a hundred various carbon- and hydrogen-based compounds known as hydrocarbons or terpenes, and each oil has its own unique combination of around a hundred different terpenes. These compounds allow every plant to create an "essence" with unique biological activity and properties that can directly affect a person's well-being or emotions. These oils are called "essential" and "volatile," where both words refer to the same plant-derived liquid, because of the volatile nature essential oils have due to their ability to vaporize.

Because oils are made of hundreds of different constituents, and environmental conditions are constantly changing, **no two batches of oils are *exactly* the same.**

A Brief History

From all the records available, it seems that the Egyptians were the first people to use aromatic herbs and essential oils for religious as well as medicinal purposes. They are thought to have developed the distillation method which is still used to extract essential oils today. This system was passed down until it reached the Peruvian physician named *Avicenna* who is credited for perfecting it in approximately 1000 AD.

Since then, usage of them has dipped in and out of fashion. For example, in the Dark Ages, it was considered witchcraft, but these days, aromatherapy and alternative medications are *extremely* popular. That's because people are becoming increasingly inclined to heal themselves in a way that avoids all of the toxins and negative side effects of traditional medication.

Below is an *Aromatherapy Timeline*:

Cave paintings in Lascaux, France testify to the use of aromatic plants in primitive societies as far back as 18,000 BC. Beginning in the mystery of religious ritual, people have long valued fragrances for their spiritual, cleansing, and pleasurable effects.

7000-4000 BC

Neolithic ointments were made by infusing fragrant plant material with Sesame and Olive oils and used to anoint the body for religious ceremonies or for cosmetic use. Herbs were also often thrown on tribal fires for their narcotic effects on the mind.

3000 BC

Ancient Egyptian papyri dating back to 3000 BC record the import of large quantities of herbs and spices primarily for use as religious ointments in the Indus Valley, a terra cotta still was built along with terra cotta perfume pots.

2650 BC

During the reign of Emperor Huang Ti, or the Yellow Emperor as he was known, a treatise on herbal medicine and massage was published called *The Yellow Emperor's Classic of Internal Medicine*. It explains the use of many aromatic plants.

2500 BC

The Egyptians perfected their secret art of perfumery. A temple wall in Denderah reveals a method of oil extraction that is still used by Egyptian farmers today. Perfume was of immense spiritual importance to the Egyptian society.

2000 BC

Around this time, a vessel of similar design to the still built in the Indus Valley was being constructed in Afghanistan. Both these findings suggest that essential oils were available to people some 4,000 years earlier than first believed.

1700 BC

The Middle East was the hub of established trading routes for fragrant goods carried from Gilead to Egypt by the Ishmaelites (Arabs). The Old Testament mentions products such as "spicery, balms and myrrh going to carry it down to Egypt."

1200 BC

The Book of Exodus records how the Jews took too much knowledge of herbs and spices with them as they fled from Egypt. A recipe for anointing oil was given to Moses; it blended together Myrrh, Cinnamon, Calamus, and Olive oils.

800-700 BC

Corinthian, Rhodian, and eastern Greek traders dominated trade in perfume flasks and containers for makeup. The Greeks also invaded Egypt around this time to obtain their great medical and scientific knowledge of aromatics.

500-400 BC

Babylon became the height of the perfume trade in the late 5th century BC, and among the plants they used were: cypress, pine, fir, resin, myrtle, calamus, and juniper. Babylonians used scents more in the way of incenses than essential oils.

300-100 BC

Persian traders brought myrrh and frankincense from Yemen to the

Mediterranean and soon demand grew for roses, saffron, spikenard, ginger, and many other aromatics. The Romans were particularly hedonistic in their use of fragrance.

100 AD

The 1st century AD was a time of great progress for aromatherapy. About 2800 tons of frankincense were imported to Rome per year, and Pliny's *Natural History* includes 32 flower remedies. The *New Testament* refers to many herbs, and Gnostic Christians valued the spirituality of fragrances.

400-500 AD

With the Roman Empire in decline, Europe began its descent into the Dark Ages. The Christian church forbade the personal use of essential oils, and knowledge of medicinal plants became confined to religious ceremonies. But progress continued in the East.

500-600 AD

The Chinese upper class were almost as lavish as the Romans, scenting their baths, bodies, homes, and temples. By 500 AD, the Japanese had already set up an effective distillation process. Meanwhile, the spread of Islam helped preserve the ancient knowledge of aromatics.

800-900 AD

Arab alchemists studied, translated and found their essential oils represented the true nature of plants. Yakub al-Kindi's *The Book of Perfume Chemistry and Distillation* gives details of many essential oils, including Chinese Camphor.

930-1037 AD

During his lifetime Avicenna wrote around 100 books and devoted one book to roses. He is often credited with inventing distillation, though now it appears that he greatly improved upon a process the ancient world had already discovered. And he made much use of essential oils in his practice.

1200-1400 AD

Thanks to the famous perfumes of Arabia and the Crusades, aromatherapy had returned to Europe by this era. The spice trade proved highly profitable, shipping spices and herbs to plague-ridden cities. Skirmishes over popular spice trading routes were common.

1500-1600 AD

The Renaissance revitalized aromatherapy with imports from the East; explorer merchants brought back exotic wares of new herbs and oils to add to the European Herbalists repertoire. Fragrance became more popular again to scent wigs and handkerchiefs.

1700-1800 AD

Herbalists of the 16th and 17th centuries, such as Nicholas Culpeper, happily married medical herbalism with everyday wisdom. Culpeper, specifically, is known for his work to make medical knowledge available to everyone, rather than being hidden within Latin texts.

1900 AD

French chemist Gattefosse's accidental discovery of Lavender oil's healing power led to scientific research into the therapeutic properties of essential oils; he also coined the phrase 'aromatherapy.' Later, Marguerite Maury combines essential oil chemistry with beauty therapy and massage.

2000 AD

Many self-regulating aromatherapy organizations exist today, and in France, the birth place of modern aromatherapy, essential oils are available to everyone to buy. Some doctors will even prescribe essential oils to patients.

2 WAYS ESSENTIAL OILS WORK

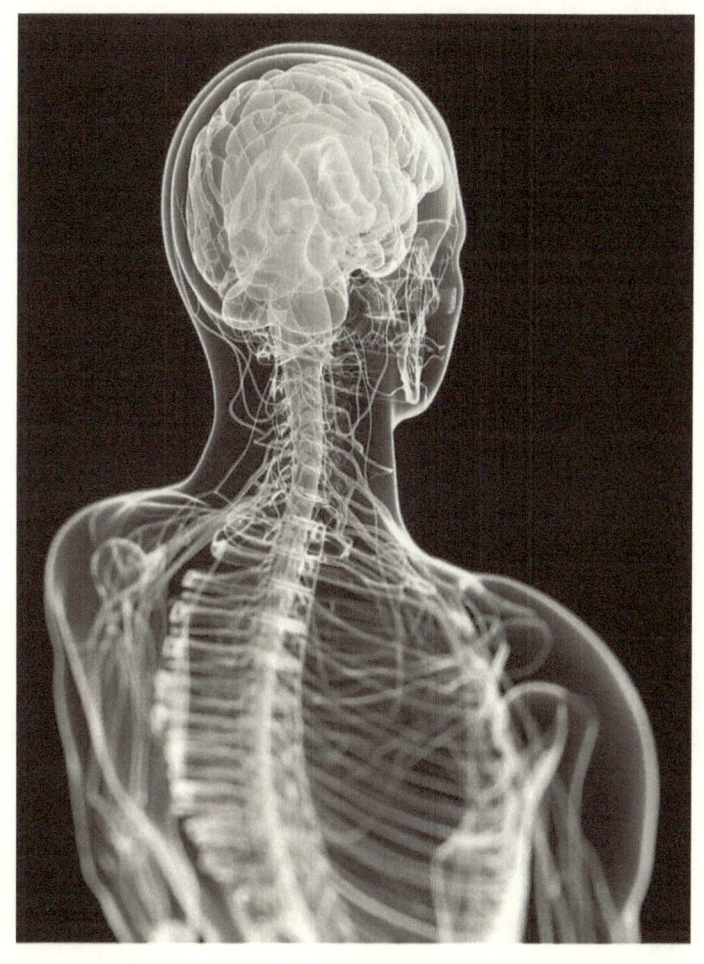

There are 2 ways in which essential oils work on your body. This is through body chemistry and the nervous system. Knowing exactly *how* these essentials oils get into – and start to work on – your body, can give you a better idea of exactly what they're doing, and how effective they are for therapeutic purposes.

1.   *Our Body Chemistry*

Every plant extract has unique biological properties, and after essential oils are absorbed into the body, they work directly with our chemistry to impact specific systems or issues, such as reducing inflammation or rejuvenating cells. The lung membranes, skin pores, and hair follicles easily absorb the chemical compounds of the essential oils that are then carried into the bloodstream to every area of our bodies. Essential oils are a natural way to generate gentle physiological change within your body.

2.   *The Nervous System*

Essential oils offer a sense of healing that works on the mental and emotional levels. Psychological benefits can be better obtained if essential oils are applied through inhalation. A person's sense of smell is activated by an organ at the top of the nose, which is home to the cilia and receptor cells that speak directly to the brain. Inhaling that aroma will send a clear message to the limbic system, which is where we retain memories and emotions. A variety of oils will have a strong effect on your mind, moods, and emotions.

ULTIMATE REASONS
TO USE THEM

Essential oils can be absorbed into the body in these three ways:

- Spread directly on the skin
- Ingest on food or in drinks
- Inhale through nose and mouth

Only *very* experienced essential oil users should ingest the oils! The most popular method of application for beginners is topical and inhalation.

Inhalation: To best affect our minds and bodies, this can be the most direct application method for the incredibly healing components in essential oils, because the nasal cavity and its receptor cells have immediate access to the brain.

How the Body Responds to Essential Oils Through Inhalation

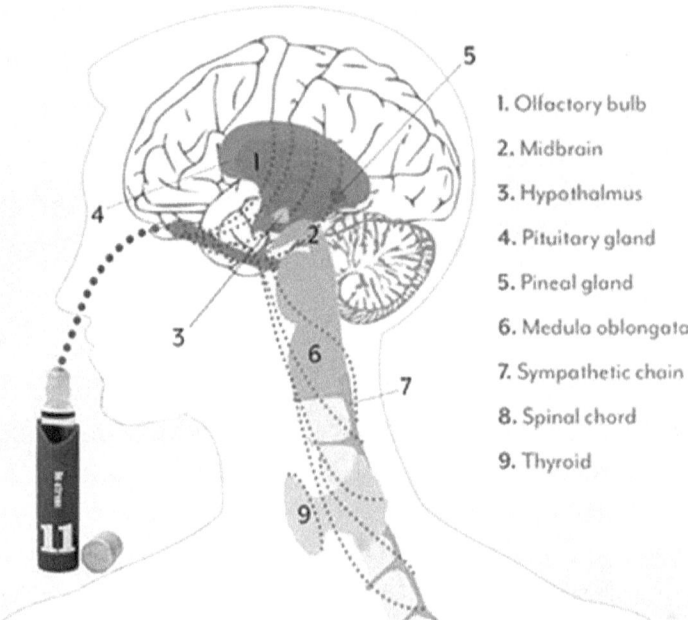

1. Olfactory bulb
2. Midbrain
3. Hypothalmus
4. Pituitary gland
5. Pineal gland
6. Medula oblongata
7. Sympathetic chain
8. Spinal chord
9. Thyroid

Topical: Applying essential oils directly to the skin allows their healing components to be absorbed by hair follicles and pores, which leads them right into the bloodstream. Once there, they can spread out to specific organs and systems where their work is needed. Focus on your body's pulse points. These are areas on your body where the blood vessels are closest to your skin's surface. Applying essential oils there allows them to work more quickly and be absorbed faster. The back of your neck, inner wrists, and temples are optimal spots.

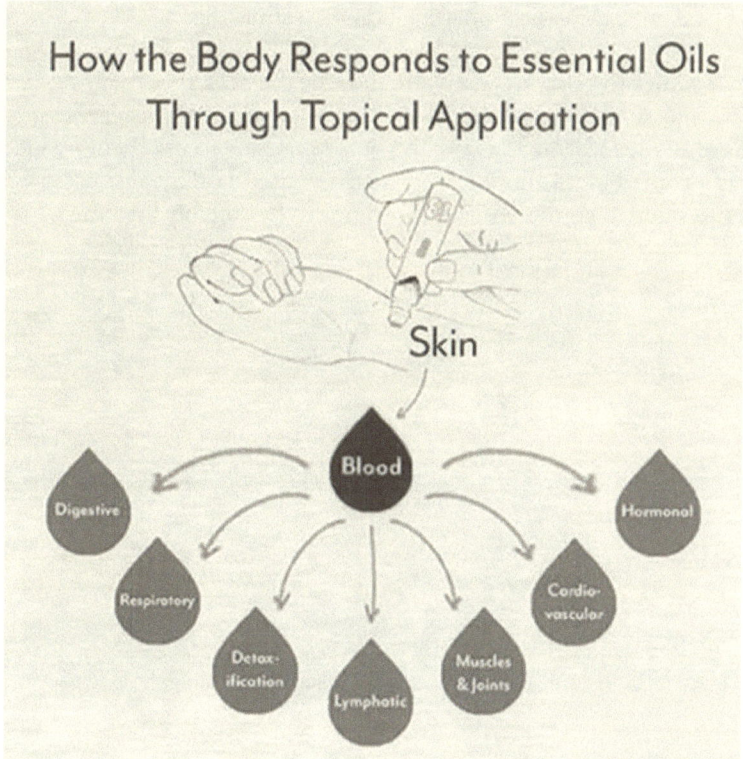

How the Body Responds to Essential Oils Through Topical Application

Many studies have been conducted by companies to discover the true benefits of these home remedies. The list of the **Top Benefits found** is:

1. They aren't toxic, so are extremely **safe** to use (if used correctly).
2. They are much **easier** to use than traditional medicine.
3. You can administer them **anywhere**, even at home.
4. They can **travel** with you everywhere you go.
5. They can be used to **cure or prevent** anything (almost)!

Of course, there are also some **negative points when it comes to essential oils**, and these must be considered too when making the choice to use them. The most prominent are:

- There isn't the same *regulation* as traditional medicine.

- *Limited research* – although there is more being conducted all the time.

- As with all medication, the *side effects* can vary so it's best to be aware of this. It is always advisable to speak to a health professional before taking *any* medication – including essential oils.

When it comes to using essential oils, most of the negative effects or mistakes are down to simple errors and lack of knowledge, so it's best to ensure that you have all the information on hand before starting to use them. Aside from what is included in this book, there are many useful online resources when it comes to safety – so there is no reason not to be suitably informed.

15 THINGS YOU DIDN'T KNOW ABOUT ESSENTIAL OILS

When it comes to essential oil usage, there *are* some things you'll need to know; here is a very interesting list for you:

1. **Essential oils won't feel oily**. Plants generate two oil types: vegetable oils, typically made up (greasy) fatty acids and triglycerides, and essential oils, which, as previously stated, are made up of (non-greasy) volatile compounds.

2. **Essential oils have more than one chemical element**. Most essential oils contain one, two, or three major elements, where each element can comprise about 20-90% of the oil's whole makeup. A couple minor constituents could comprise about 1-19% each, while several more could comprise less than 1% each.

3. **No two essential oils are the same**. Several different factors can have an impact when it comes to the makeup of an essential oil. A single constituent's percentage often changes from one harvest to another. That's just one reason that testing an oil before use is so important. There is a great potential for contaminants, dilutions, or adulterating substances, which depends on how the plant is grown, harvested, and how the oil is extracted and processed.

4. **Essential oils are extracted with multiple methods**. Steam distillation, cold pressing (or expression, to extract citrus oils), and hydro distillation are just a couple. Absolutes and CO_2 extracts are two additional types of natural aromatic extracts.

5. **Large quantities of source plants are required to extract essential oils**. In the case of Rose essential oil, it is reported that roughly

60,000 roses are needed to extract only 1 ounce of oil.

6. **Oxidation can reduce quality of some essential oils**. Oxidation is caused by light, heat, air, and moisture interacting with stored oils and can adversely affect the oil's composition. Always storing your oils in a tightly capped, dark glass bottle is the best way to avoid this. You could potentially double your oils' effective lifespans (in some cases beyond 7-10 years) by keeping your essential oils refrigerated.

7. **To be safe, dilute most essential oils before use**. There will be more information about dilution in this book.

8. **Avoid ingesting essential oils on a daily basis**. It is recommended that you only use these oils as needed and not simply because they are available to you.

9. **Practice extra caution with essential oils when pregnant women and young children seek use**. This book will clearly discuss the essential oils that should ALWAYS be avoided during pregnancy. It is recommended for pregnant women and young children that dilution starts at 0.5%. Increase to 3% only if needed and after considering the child's age and type of oil.

10. **Inhaling through mouth or nose is typically the best way to apply essential oils**. Some of the ways to do this is via diffusion, by including a few drops in bath water or on the floor of your shower, and by applying the oils to the back of your neck or chest. Note: topical use is best for wounds or other skin issues.

11. **Essential oils have also been known to offer assistance with or relief from**: killing fungus, viruses, and bacteria; boosting the immune system; alleviating nausea, inflammation, congestion, pain, headaches, memory loss, and more concerns.

12. **The FDA's GRAS rating for some essential oils**. The FDA has stated that some essential oils are Generally Regarded as Safe. Note, though, that no government agency certifies or provides grades for essential oils. Therapeutic-grade, Certified Pure Therapeutic-Grade, and pharmaceutical grade are agreed upon terms that are used within the current oil industry. Avoid buying essential oils without considering factors beyond their grade or certification. When you buy essential oils, be sure to research and thoroughly understand industry tests or know and trust the company selling the oils you seek. Take into consideration how willing the company is to give you answers to your essential oil questions.

13. **Take note of this important information when you buy an essential oil**. Research and keep track of the botanical name, country or region of plant's origin (which can change the percentages for

chemical constituents), extraction method, and chemotype (where applicable). Even when it is a natural dilution, be sure to note when the essential oil has been diluted and with what.

14. **Combined properly, essential oils can have more therapeutic power**. When essential oils are blended, these combinations are called synergies. This combination brings together essential oils that are similar in chemical families and therapeutic properties.

15. **Essential oils *need* to be tested**. Conducting tests, such as GC/MS testing, on essential oils will reveal the quality of the oil's purity and the percentages of its constituents. A smell test could also be performed, where trained experts can determine if an oil is pure or adulterated with a single sniff. A drip or two on a test strip, at different timed intervals, will allow the tester to discern among the oil's top, middle, and base notes.

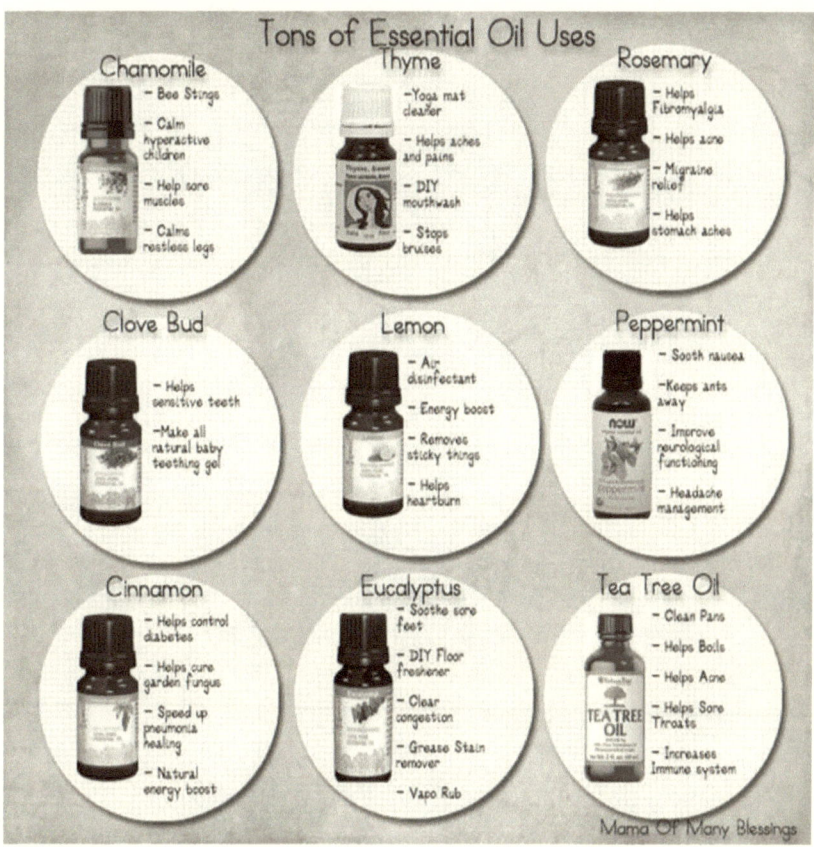

PROVEN STEPS FOR BUYING ESSENTIAL OILS

There will come a time when you will want to buy your own essential oils. While health professionals and experts *will* be able to help you, it is always best to be armed with your own knowledge to start with – to ensure that you're more likely to get *exactly* what you want.

When you start buying essential oils, there are a **few things you will want to consider**:

1. ***Why*** do you want the essential oil? What is it for?
2. Consider ***what grade*** of oil you want (guidelines for this below).
3. ***Learn everything*** you need to know ***about the oil*** in question – knowledge is power.
4. ***Shop around*** – there are a number of companies out there, so discover all you can about their reputation and how they do business. Any question you have, just ask them!
5. ***Look at pricing***, but bear in mind more expensive doesn't always mean better. The "Pure vs. Quality" chapter below covers this in more detail.

Knowing about the oil grades is extremely useful – especially when you're considering them for their healing properties. As there is currently no regulating body for these oils, this **grade chart** has been created to help buyers know exactly what it is they're getting. Note, that no government agency or organization has formally approved "grades" or "certifications" for essential oils, such as "therapeutic grade," "medicinal grade," or "aromatherapy grade," within the United States. In fact, the entire industry lacks a consistent grading standard, so the chart below is only provided for informational purposes.

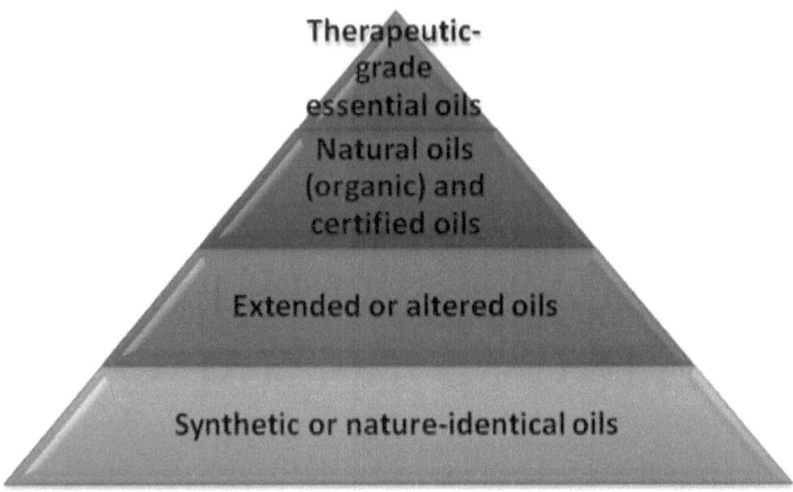

Therapeutic-grade essential oils	Pure, medicinal, steam-distilled essential oils containing all desired therapeutic compounds
Natural oils (organic) and certified oils	Pass oil-standard tests but may not contain any or just a few therapeutic compounds
Extended or altered oils	Fragrance grade
Synthetic or nature-identical oils	Created in a laboratory

For what we are looking at here, therapeutic-grade oils are the most common ones you'll be looking at. The recommendation is to **look out for 100% therapeutic-grade** essential oils wherever possible. Just be aware and keep in mind that, even though such terms can mislead, companies are not using those words to intentionally deceive you.

Many factors are considered when producing therapeutic-grade essential oils, but overall, they can be organized into two categories.

Physical Factors – How source plants are harvested, oils are extracted or distilled, and oils are stored or bottled.

Environmental Factors – Where source plants are grown, quality of the soil, and use of chemical or organic fertilizers.

These therapeutic-grade oils meet stringent distillation and testing procedures and are produced with no solvents. They are costly to produce, which means there aren't many high-quality producers, but a little research will lead you to a reputable company. When you notice a company that employs descriptions such as *aromatherapy grade* or *therapeutic grade*, make it a point to look at additional factors that will indicate the quality of an essential oil. Try to assess the company's intent when they use that particular term. While there are companies using those words in a way that misleads or intentionally deceives, most companies will provide clear details that explain why they use that particular term.

Top Essential Oil Brands

There are many brands of essential oils on the market, but the most popular brands are:

Young Living at www.youngliving.org

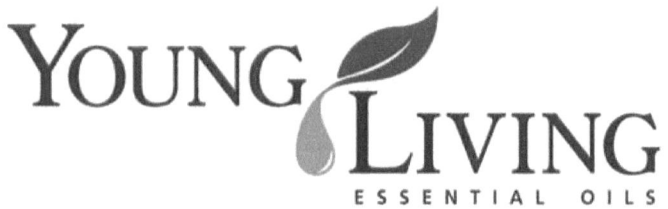

"Through the painstaking steps of our proprietary Seed to Seal production process, we produce the best, most authentic essential oils in the world. We are committed to providing pure, powerful products for every family and lifestyle, all infused with the life-changing benefits of our essential oils."

Although they are one of the most expensive essential oil companies in the marketplace, it's well worth the price, because they have the largest inventory of 100% pure therapeutic-grade essential oils and they've been in business since 1993.

Eden's Garden at www.edensgarden.com

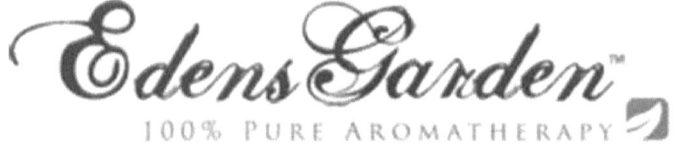

"Our philosophy is pretty simple. At Edens Garden, we believe that everyone deserves a break. Today's busy world can take its toll even on the best multi-tasker or superior planner. Our goal is to create life-giving moments for our customers. Everyone deserves to dip their toes in the sand, sip tea with friends or slip into the tub with a good book. And that's why we offer the very best pure essential oils at affordable, practical prices."

Edens Garden offers over 150 essential oils and a lot of discounts, deals, and bonuses. The company controls product quality with a two-week rotation of their stock to maintain freshness. The oils are 100% therapeutic-grade.

DoTerra at www.doterra.com

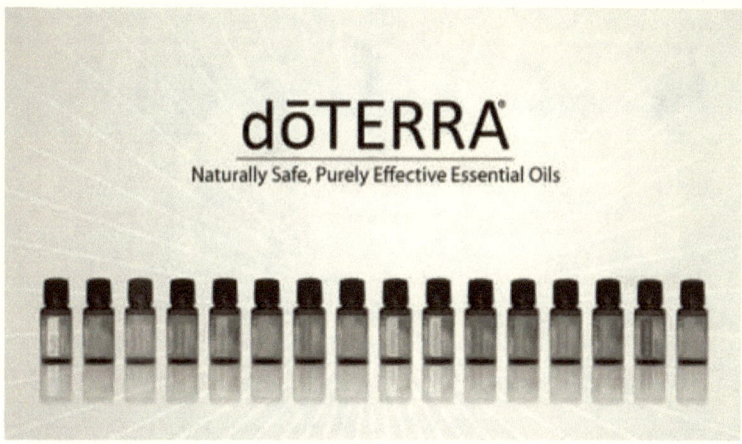

"dōTerra, meaning 'gift of the Earth' in Latin, came to life with the intention of introducing to market CPTG Certified Pure Therapeutic Grade® essential oils, a quality standard more pure and potent than anything that existed previously."

They have been operating since 2008, and they use CPTG (Certified Pure Therapeutic Grade) testing for oil purity. Because they don't maintain their own farms for growing source plants, their products are less expensive than the Young Living company's products.

Plant Therapy at www.planttherapy.com

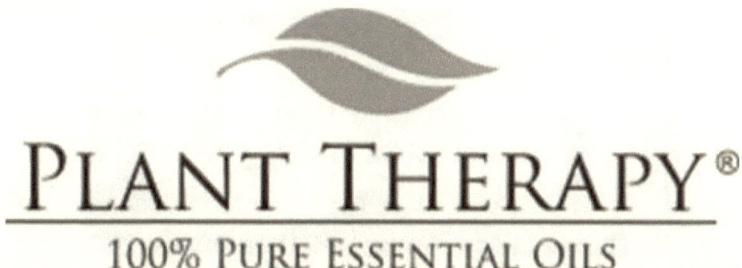

This family-owned company has been operating out of Idaho since 2011. They offer 100% pure, undiluted essential oils. These quality oils are provided by premier suppliers from all over the world. Employing their own team of experts, Plant Therapy® performs or oversees third-party testing to monitor GC/MS processes. Despite not having their own farms to grow source plants, they insist on acquiring oils from top suppliers and offering only the best customer support.

Aura Cacia at www.auracacia.com

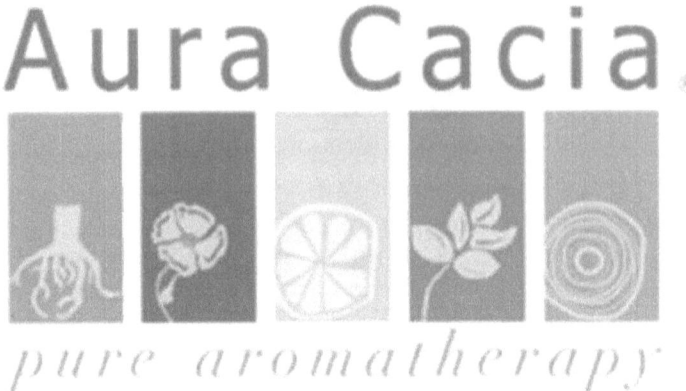

"At Aura Cacia, our goal is to make aromatherapy easy! We offer an extensive selection of high-quality essential oils and aromatherapy products for all ages and spaces."

This company began in 1982 and is a leader in 100% pure essential oils. Their oils are sourced from Oregon, Europe, Ukraine, and Australia. Moreover, their products are priced at competitive prices and are highly available in major food stores.

NOW Foods Essential Oils at www.nowfoods.com/Personal-Care/Products/Aromatherapy

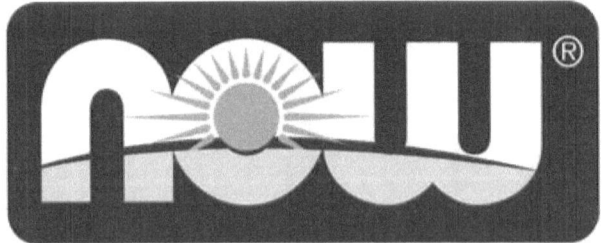

Nutrition for Optimal Wellness™

"The integrity of an essential oil is determined by the botanical from which it was derived, proper harvest and gentle extraction methods to bring products to life."

Operating out of Chicago, Illinois, NOW founded this natural foods and supplements business in 1948. All of their oils are distilled using a unique technique: growing specific source plants, then harvesting and distilling them to prepare pure essential oils of the highest quality that are only grown during a certain season. However, they do not apply any official grading (A, B, C, or therapeutic) to their products.

Native American Nutritionals at www.nativeamericannutritionals.com

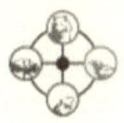 Native American Nutritionals

"Our company is founded upon integrity and the desire to guide people on their journey to good health by providing the best therapeutic quality essential oils, supplements and other products from earth's bounty."

This company truly cares about alternative methods for healing and offers single species plants that are grown on small organic farms. Note: their oils tend to have a thin consistency, which can make it difficult to get an accurate number of drops.

Mountain Rose Herbs at www.mountainroseherbs.com

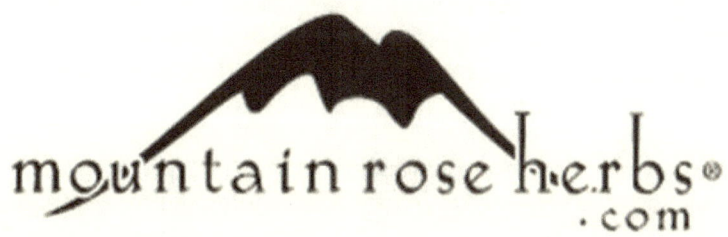

"Mountain Rose Herbs offers high quality organic bulk herbs, gourmet spices, loose leaf teas, essential oils, herbal extracts, and natural body care ingredients. Our extensive selection includes certified organic, fair trade, ethically wild harvested, & Kosher certified botanical products."

The company has produced essential oils since 1987. They provide therapeutic-grade essential oils and have a wide range of reasonably priced products.

Healing Solutions Essential Oils at healingsolutions.com

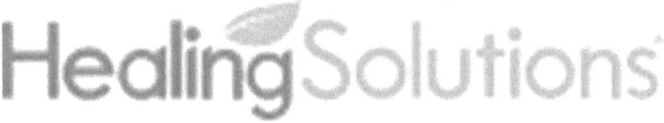

Healing Solutions operates out of Arizona and offers only premium essential oils. They sell products directly on Amazon, which helps to keep the prices low. They offer more than 170 different oils to use alone or blend, and their customer support is superior.

Rocky Mountain Oils at www.rockymountainoils.com

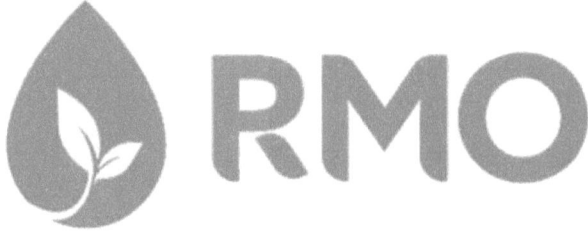

Rocky Mountain Oils began operations in 2004. They obtain their oils from small organic farms all over the world. These essential oils are classified 100% pure, therapeutic-grade. They offer more than 100 singles and 75 blends of quality products. Note that the company offers a full refund after a 90-day guarantee on oils if the product doesn't meet your expectations.

Of course, you will have to do some research and experimentation to see which brand you prefer – every individual has different needs, likes, and desires, so it's impossible to predict which will be your personal favorite.

It is important to remember that essential oils can cost anything from a couple of dollars to 50+ dollars. The price isn't *necessarily* a guide to how good the product is. You are much more likely to get a better picture of this by researching the company's reputation. There are a lot of online forum and review sites that can assist you with this.

10 Tricks You Should Know Before You Buy

Below is a great list of buying tips available for you that have come from real consumers. Read through the list of ten below and keep them in mind when you're buying your own.

- Use the smell test for different oil brands by holding the lid at least 5 inches away from your nose and then inhaling.
- Take breaks while performing the smell test. Inhaling a variety of oils back to back will overwhelm the senses. This hinders your ability to notice the differences among oils.
- Different oils should not be given the same prices. This could be a sign of synthetic or lower quality essential oils. Prices should vary according to the quantity of source material required to extract or distill the oil.
- Test for essential oils that have been diluted with vegetable oils. Perform this test by placing a couple drops of an essential oil in the middle of a slip of paper to see if an oily stain remains. Stop use immediately.
- Rely on essential oil companies that provide each oil's Latin name alongside the common name, country of origin, and method of extraction.
- Look for pure essential oils rather than synthetic oils. Aromatherapists make this suggestion, noting that synthetics may not have similar therapeutic properties.
- Be sure that you see "pure essential oil" or "100% essential oil" printed clearly on a label before you purchase.
- Even if you see the words "pure essential oil," this says nothing about the oil's physical factors such as how the plant was grown or how the oil was stored.
- Look for essential oils sold in bottles that are dark amber or blue glass. Clear glass will allow light to affect the oil and cause it to spoil.
- Essential oils should never be sold in plastic bottles. The bottles can dissolve and then contaminate the essential oil.

Pure vs. Quality

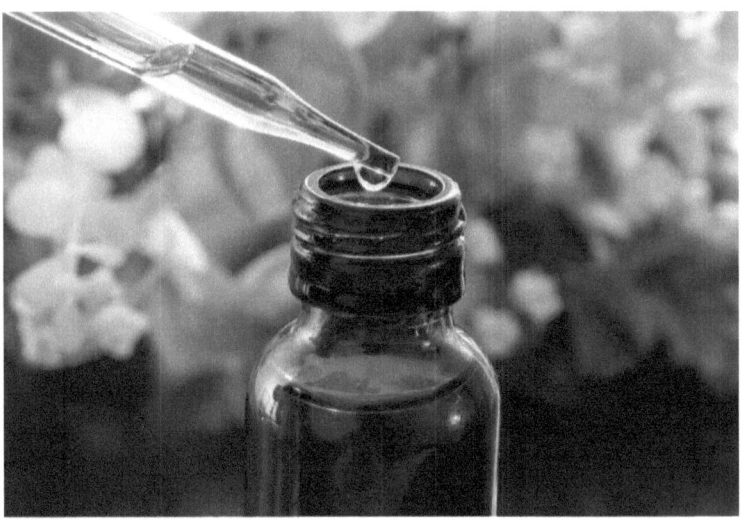

As stated before, it is also important to know **the difference between '*pure*' and '*quality*'** essential oils when buying. Pure means undiluted, whereas quality refers to how well the product is made. There can be a bad quality oil that's pure. For more information about pure and quality oils, check out the NAHA website at www.nha.org.

It may surprise you to learn that **large quantities of source plants are required to extract essential oil**. In fact, 1 drop of Peppermint essential oil is equal to 26 cups of peppermint tea. This just shows how much work and material is needed to make this, which is why a number of people believe that the higher the price of the product, the better the quality will be (but just to reiterate, quality is not to be confused with 'pure').

You could also do a little research into a company's standards and reputation and make a judgment on the quality of the oil for yourself. The choice is yours to make, but it's always recommended to discuss anything you use with a health professional or expert.

So now that you know the oil grade that you need and the difference between 'pure' and 'quality,' it's time to focus on the actual product required. Of course, that entirely depends on the ailment you – or your loved one – is suffering from, so we will go into detail on a variety of different scenarios – so you're bound to find something specific to you!

12 LITTLE KNOWN FACTS ABOUT ESSENTIAL OILS

Here are some little-known facts about the benefits of pure, therapeutic-grade essential oils:

1. The immune defense, oxygenating, and regenerating properties of plants are contained in their essential oils.

2. An essential oil's smaller molecular constituents can quickly penetrate the skin's pores and hair follicles.

3. Essential oils can affect every cell of the body within 20 minutes and can penetrate cell walls, even after being hardened by oxygen deficiency. They are lipid soluble and can be metabolized just like any other nutrient.

4. Essential oils can help transport nutrients to starving body cells because they contain oxygen molecules. This work stimulates the immune system, to the point where essential oils can prevent the beginning of disease by providing needed oxygen where there is a nutritional deficiency due to a lack of proper assimilation.

5. Essential oils work against free radicals as effective antioxidants. They scavenge free radicals and prevent mutations, fungus, and cellular oxidation.

6. Essential oils are known to destroy viruses and bacteria and bring much needed balance to your body. They are antiseptic, antibacterial, antiviral, antifungal, antimicrobial, anti-infectious, antiparasitic, anti-tumoral, and anticancerous.

7. The human body's cells and blood can be detoxified by essential oils.

8. Some essential oils are effective in treating Parkinson's disease, Lou Gehrig's disease, multiple sclerosis, and Alzheimer's disease because they contain sesquiterpenes, which can pass the blood brain barrier.

9. Essential oils not only fill the air with a fresh scent, they can perform air purification. They are considered aromatic, and when diffused, they purify by eradicating mold, cigarette, and animal odors; enhancing atmospheric oxygen, ozone, and negative ions, which hinders bacterial growth; and eliminating toxins and metallic particles from the air.

10. Essential oils support spiritual, physical, and emotional healing.

11. Essential oils exhibit a bio-electrical frequency that can directly impact the human body's frequency, even bring it back to a normal, healthy level. This inherent frequency is several times greater than that found in herbs, food, or even the human body itself.

12. There is a great test so that you can discover if your essential oils are pure at home:

   Apply a single drop of essential oil to a piece of construction paper. If it evaporates, leaving no noticeable ring, it is pure. If a ring remains, it has most likely been diluted with another kind of oil. This test doesn't work with patchouli, myrrh, and absolutes.

A QUICK REFERENCE GUIDE TO BOTANICAL NAMES

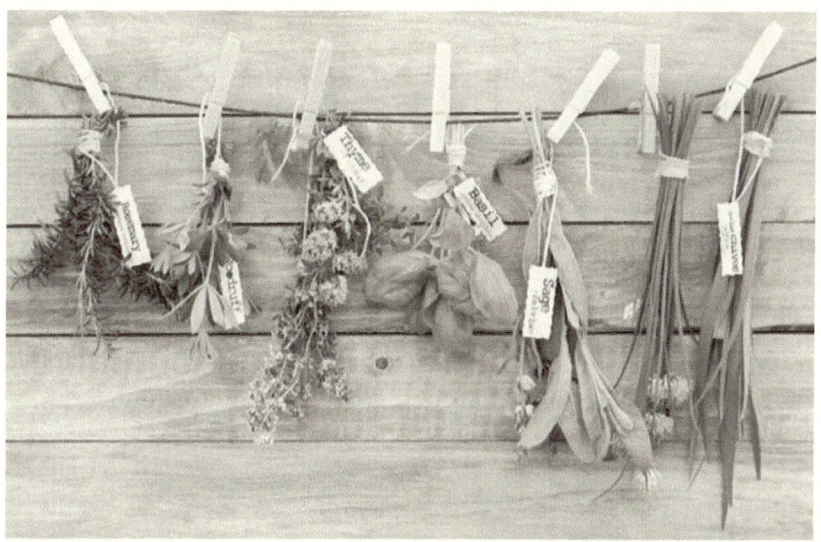

Many experts in the use of essential oils suggest that you have a much better chance of buying the best quality possible if you have a good knowledge of the botanical names associated with ingredients. You can keep the chart below as a reference guide to ensure you're constantly in the know.

Oil	Botanical Name
Ambrette Seed	*Hibiscus abelmoschus*
Angelica	*Angelica archangelica*
Anise	*Pimpinella anisum*
Atlas Cedar	*Cedrus atlantica*
Balsam Copaiba	*Copaifera officinalis*
Balsam Peru	*Myroxylon pereirae*
Balsam Tolu	*Myroxylon balsamum*
Bay Laurel	*Laurus nobilis*
Basil	*Ocimum basilicum var.Linalool*
Benzoin	*Styrax benzoin*
Bergamot	*Citrus bergamia*
Bergamot Mint	*Mentha citrate*
Black Pepper	*Piper nigrum*
Blue Tansy	*Tanacetum annuum*
Camphor White	*Cinnamomum camphora (Bark)*
Cardamom	*Elettaria cardamomum*
Carrot	*Daucua carota*
Cassia	*Cinnamomum cassia*
Cedar Red	*Thuja plicata*
Cedar Leaf (Thuja)	*Thuja occidentalis*
Cedarwood (Atlas Cedar)	*Cedrus atlantica*

Chamomile Cape	*Eriocephalus punctulatus*
Chamomile German (Blue)	*Matricaria recutita or Chamaemelum matricaria*
Chamomile Morrocan (Blue Tansy)	*Tanacetum annuum*
Chamomile Roman	*Anthemis nobilis or Chamaemelum nobile*
Cinnamon Bark	*Cinnamomum verum*
Cinnamon Leaf	*Cinnamomum zeylanicum*
Cistus (Labdanum) (Rock Rose)	*Cistus ladaniferus*
Citronella	*Cymbopogon nardus*
Clary Sage	*Salvia sclarea*
Clove	*Syzygium aromaticum*
Cocoa	*Theobroma cacao*
Coriander	*Coriandrum savitum*
Cumin	*Cuminum cyminum*
Cypress	*Cupressus sempervirens*
Cypress Blue	*Callitris intratropica*
Davana	*Artemisia pallens*
Elemi	*Canarium luzonicum*
Eucalyptus	*Eucalyptus globules*
Eucalyptus Lemon	*Eucalyptus citriodora*
Eucalyptus Radiata	*Eucalyptus radiate*
Eucalyptus Staigeriana or Balm	*Eucalyptus Staigeriana*

Fennel	*Foeniculum vulgare*
Fir Balsam	*Abies balsamea*
Fir Silver	*Abies alba*
Fir Douglas	*Pseudotsuga menziesii*
Fir Grand	*Abies grandis*
Frankincense (Olibanum)	*Boswellia carterii or serrata or frareana*
Galbanum	*Ferula gummosa*
Geranium	*Pelargonium graveolens*
Ginger	*Zingiber officinale*
Grapefruit	*Citrus paradisii*
Helichrysum (Everlasting or Immortelle)	*Helichrysum italicum*
Hyssop	*Hyssopus officinalis*
Inula	*Inula graveolens*
Jasmine	*Jasminum officinale*
Juniper Berry	*Juniperus communis*
Khella	*Amni visnaga*
Kunzea	*Kunzea ambigua*
Lavender	*Lavandula angustifolia or officinale*
Lavendin	*Lavandula x hybrid*
Lemon	*Citrus limonum*
Lemon Myrtle	*Backhousia citriodora*
Lemon Tea Tree	*Leptospermum petersonii*

Lemon Verbena (Vervaine)	*Aloysia citriodora*
Lemongrass	*Cymbopogon flexuosus*
Lime	*Citrus aurantifolia*
Linden Blossom	*Tilia cordata*
Litsea (May Chang)	*Litsea cubeba*
Lotus White	*Nymphaea lotus*
Mandarin	*Citrus reticulata or deliciosa*
Manuka (New Zealand Tea Tree)	*Leptospermum scoparium*
Mastick	*Lentiscus pistachius*
May Chang	*Litsea cubeba*
Melissa (Lemon Balm)	*Melissa officinalis*
Marjoram	*Origanum majorana*
Mimosa	*Acacia dealbata*
Monarda (Bee Balm)	*Monarda fistulosa*
MQV (niaouli nerol type AKA Nerolina)	*Melaleuca quinquenervia veridiflora*
Myrrh	*Commiphora myrrha*
Myrtle	*Myrtus communis*
Myrtle Lemon	*Backhousia citriodora*
Neroli (Orange Blossom)	*Citrus aurantium var. Amara*
Nerolina	*Melaleuca quinquenervia veridiflora*

Niaouli	*Melaleuca quinquenervia*
Nutmeg	*Myristica fragrans*
Orange	*Citrus sinensis*
Oregano	*Origanum vulgare var.Carvacrol*
Owyhee	*Artemesia ludoviciana*
Palmarosa	*Cymbopogon martini*
Patchouli	*Pogostemon cablin*
Pepper Black	*Piper nigrum*
Peppermint	*Mentha piperita*
Petitgrain Bigarade	*Citrus aurantium var.Amara*
Pine Sylvester (Scotch Pine)	*Pinus sylvestris*
Ravensara	*Ravensara aromatic*
Ravintsara	*Cinnamomum camphora (Leaf)*
Rock Rose (Cistus) (Labdanum)	*Cistus ladaniferus*
Rosalina (Lavender Tea Tree)	*Melaleuca ericifolia*
Rose Damask (Otto)	*Rosa damascene*
Rose Moroc	*Rosa centifolia*
Rosemary	*Rosmarinus officinalis*
Rosemary Verbenone	*Rosmarinus officinalis var.Verbenon*
Rosewood	*Aniba rosaeodora*
Sage	*Salvia officinalis*

Sandalwood Australian	*Santalum spicatum*
Sandalwood Indian	*Santalum album*
Spearmint	*Mentha spicata*
Spikenard	*Nardostachys jatamansi*
Spruce Black	*Picea mariana*
St Johnswort	*Hypericum perforatum*
Tamanu (Foraha)	*Calophyllum inophyllum*
Tangerine	*Citrus reticulata or nobilis*
Tansy Blue	*Tanacetum annuum*
Tarragon	*Artemisia dracunculus*
Tea Tree	*Melaleuca alternifolia*
Tea Tree Lavender (Rosalina)	*Melaleuca ericifolia*
Tea Tree Lemon	*Leptospermum petersonii*
Tea Tree New Zealand (Manuka)	*Leptospermum scoparium*
Thyme Linalool	*Thymus vulgaris var. Linalool*
Valerian	*Valeriana officinalis*
Vanilla	*Vanilla planifolia*
Vervaine (Lemon Verbena)	*Aloysia citriodora*
Vetiver	*Vetiveria zizanoides*
Violet Leaf	*Viola odorata*
Vitex	*Vitex agnus castus*

White Lotus	*Nymphaea lotus*
Wintergreen	*Gaultheria procumbens*
Yarrow	*Achillea millefolium*
Ylang Ylang	*Cananga odorata var.Genuana*

BEST WAYS TO DILUTE ESSENTIAL OILS

Dilute, Dilute, Dilute!

LearningAboutEOs.com/dilute

Concentrated substances are rarely intended for use "as is" - and essential oils are no different. There is almost never a time when you would not want to dilute the potency of an essential oil.

Diluting essential oils is done by adding a drop (or more) of the essential oil into a carrier oil. This not only provides a good medium for the oil to absorb into the skin, but spreads the oil over a larger surface of your skin for more effect.

Another thing you need to be aware of with essential oil use is dilution. Because essential oils are *so* concentrated, they need to be diluted so that they're safe to apply. The best way to achieve this is via a '**Carrier oil.**' These carrier oils are usually derived from a plant's fatty portion, such as the seeds, nuts, or kernels. Example carrier oils include Coconut, Almond, Apricot, Olive, Macadamia, and Sesame. Store carrier oils away from light and heat to sustain freshness. Examples of these Carrier Oils are looked at in more detail later on in this chapter.

There are considered to be 5 main *distillation methods:*

Cold Pressed – This method involves pressing and grinding the fruit or seeds to extract the oil. When cold pressed, oils can maintain all of their aroma, flavor, and nutritional value.

Steam Distillation – Using the straight steam method to distill essential oils requires forcing steam through source plant material and then collecting the oil.

Water/Steam Distillation – This distillation method pushes water and steam all around and through source plant material. Then, after the steam and oils are collected, they are extracted to produce an oil.

Water Distillation – This distillation method places source plant material in boiling water. The steam and oils are collected, then extracted to produce an oil.

Solvent Extracted – Some plant aromatics are too delicate for steam distillation or too bound up in resin, so a solvent is used to make an extraction. The solvents used can be a range of substances (nontoxic and toxic) including hexane, alcohol, acetone, propane, etc. The solvent should be completely evaporated out of the finished product.

Dilution Ratios

The chart below indicates **the most effective ratios to use to dilute essential oils:**

Essential Oil Dilution Chart nourishingtreasures.com/EOdilutions						
Dilution	**1%**	**2%**	**3%**	**5%**	**10%**	**25%**
drops of EO for **1 tsp** (5ml; 1/6 oz.) carrier oil	1	2	3	5	10	25
drops of EO for **2 tsp** (10ml; 1/3 oz.) carrier oil	2	4	6	10	20	50
drops of EO for **3 tsp** (15ml; 1/2 oz.) carrier oil	3	6	9	15	30	75
drops of EO for **4 tsp** (20ml; 2/3 oz.) carrier oil	4	8	12	20	40	100
drops of EO for **5 tsp** (25ml; 5/6 oz.) carrier oil	5	10	15	25	50	125
drops of EO for **6 tsp** (30ml; 1 oz.) carrier oil	6	12	18	30	60	150

How much to dilute really depends on the issue you want to address. Here is a handy guide to take into consideration:

Dilution Ratio	Amount	Ages	Notes
0.25%	1 drop per 4 teaspoons of carrier oil.	6 months – 6 years.	Where possible, use herbs instead for children under 2.
1%	1 dropper 1 teaspoon of carrier oil.	Ages 6+	This is also suitable for pregnant women, elderly adults, sensitive skin sufferers or people with compromised immune systems.

2%	2 drops per teaspoon of carrier oil.	Most adults.	This is a good dilution for daily skin care.
3%	3 drops per 1 teaspoon of carrier oil.	Adults.	This is best for a short-term issue. Up to 10% dilution is ok, but seek advice beforehand.
25%	25 drops per 1 teaspoon of carrier oil.	Adults.	Only occasional situations require this high a dilution – muscle cramp, bad bruising, sever pain, etc. Seek advice beforehand.
0% "Neat"	No carrier oil.	Adults.	Lavender is one of the few essential oils that can be used undiluted and only for short-term usage. Use caution and seek advice beforehand.

It is important to bear in mind that it's always **safest to use the lowest dilution possible** that gives you effective results. Overdosing is an issue that is easily avoided by following this rule:

The higher the percentage of EO on your skin (i.e. "neat" being highest), the higher the chance of a reaction and risk.

– Robert Tisserand

Top 10 Carrier Oils

So as you've seen, carrier oils are used to dilute absolutes and essential oils before being applied directly to the skin for use in massage therapy and aromatherapy. They are given this name because they "carry" the essential oil so it is safe to use on your skin. Some carrier oils, such as Olive, will produce a mild distinctive aroma, but most will not have as strong of an aroma as essential oils. Select carrier oils that are as natural and unadulterated as possible. If you can find organic oils, many people find them to be of higher quality. Two methods used to extract carrier oils are cold pressing and maceration.

Choosing the appropriate carrier oil will depend on your health conditions, sensitivity levels and requirements, and the area that's being massaged. A variety of carrier oils offer any number of therapeutic properties. *Considering massage?* Viscosity will be a major selling point. Note: Olive oil is typically very thick, whereas Grapeseed oil is much thinner. Sweet Almond and Sunflower oils provide viscosities that fall between those extremes. Blend carrier oils to combine ideal properties, such as aroma, lubrication, viscosity, and absorption.

The following **10 carrier oils are suggested to be the best** for use with essential oils:

- **Organic Apricot Kernel Oil**: Appropriate for any skin type; particularly benefits dry, sensitive, prematurely aged, and inflamed skin.

- **Organic Avocado Oil**: This pure, therapeutic quality, certified organic oil is a popular heavy massage oil. This oil helps to support softer and smoother skin and provides benefits for people living with psoriasis, eczema, and other skin conditions.

- **Superior Organic, Cold-Pressed Coconut Oil**: This pure, therapeutic quality, certified organic oil is popular across the globe. Coconut oil provides protection from the elements, enhancing its use as a skin moisturizer.

- **Organic Grapeseed Oil**: This general-purpose oil is virtually odorless when refined, but when cold pressed, it bears a distinctive, slightly acidic aroma. Grapeseed oil has a smooth, silky texture, which can be quickly absorbed into the skin without leaving a greasy residue.

- **Organic Extra Virgin Olive Oil**: One of the most universally used oils for hair care products, cosmetics, and food preparation. This carrier oil has been applied in virtually every skin-care product, treating everything from dehydrated skin to acne.

- **Peach Kernel Oil**: This pure, therapeutic quality oil is good for all types of skin, also for dry, flaky, cracked, sensitive, and mature skin types.

- **Organic Sesame Oil**: This oil is popular in Ayurvedic massage and is often applied due to its many helpful qualities. For example, it is a warming oil, so it is highly recommended for people who have poor circulation.

- **Organic, Cold-Pressed Jojoba Oil**: This oil is great for hair, skin, nails, and more. People suffering from acne conditions will benefit from this non-greasy oil that contains anti-inflammatory properties. It's a perfect moisturizer for all skin types and great for such skin conditions as psoriasis, eczema, sunburn, and chapped skin.

- **Sweet Almond Oil**: One of the most popular carrier oils in aroma-therapy massage. It suits most skin types and moves easily over the skin. It has fantastic moisturizing properties such as Vitamins B and E, nutrients, minerals and is a rich source of monounsaturated fats.

- **Rosehip Seed Oil**: This luxurious natural skin-care product is best used for aging skin. Its smoothing property is said to help reduce wrinkles.

5 ULTIMATE STEPS FOR BLENDING ESSENTIAL OILS

When you become confident in the use of essential oils, there may come a time when you want to create your own. There is an entire chapter in this book with recipes for essential oils to help with common ailments, so you can give this a go if you so choose.

Here is a great step-by-step guide to blending essential oils:

Step 1 – Know Which Properties You Need

You can do this with a little bit of research. The internet is a great way to do this; simply use search terms such as 'revitalizing essential oils,' and you'll find many resources letting you know what you need.

Step 2 – Blend Oils Based on Notes and Categories

Beginners often struggle with this part, but with a little bit of practice, you will quickly come to grips with what needs to be done. You will need to become familiar with the essential oil categories – a term which is used to help you get a great smell with your blended essential oils.

Essential oils categories are based on inherent aromas, where oils within the same categories are more likely to blend well together. Feel free to mix and match, though, as shown below:

- *Floral*
  (i.e. Lavender, Neroli, Jasmine)
- *Woodsy*
  (i.e. Pine, Cedar)

- *Earthy*
  (i.e. Oakmoss, Vetiver, Patchouli)

- *Herbaceous*
  (i.e. Marjoram, Rosemary, Basil)

- *Minty*
  (i.e. Peppermint, Spearmint)

- *Medicinal/Camphorous*
  (i.e. Eucalyptus, Cajuput, Tea Tree)

- *Spicy*
  (i.e. Nutmeg, Clove, Cinnamon)

- *Oriental*
  (i.e. Ginger, Patchouli)

- *Citrus*
  (i.e. Orange, Lemon, Lime)

There is also a suggestion of which of these **categories blend well together**:

- *Floral* oils will blend with spicy and *citrusy* oils.

- *Woodsy* oils will typically blend with every category.

- *Minty* oils will blend with citrus, *herbaceous*, and *earthy* oils.

- *Spicy* and *oriental* oils will blend with *florals*, *citrus*, and *oriental* oils. Note: use oriental or spicy oils with care; it is easy to overpower a blend with them.

Another term you will become very familiar with is the *'Note'* of an essential oil. The level of an oil's note is determined by how fast it evaporates. Right after applying a blend of oils to your skin, it will carry one aroma, but a short time later, it will smell another way. This is because one or more of the oils in that blend will have evaporated. These notes are known as top, middle, and base notes.

Perfume 101

top notes	middle notes	base notes
wild orange	geranium	sandalwood
jasmine	lemongrass	frankincense
bergamot	clary sage	patchouli
grapefruit	juniper berry	myrrh
lemon	melissa	ylang ylang
coriander	lavender	cassia
rose	marjoram	cedarwood
lime	rosemary	cinnamon
peppermint	cypress	vetiver
basil	black pepper	ginger

Most times, for beginners, it's recommended that you only *start with three oils*. A top note oil, a middle note oil, and a base note oil (for example: bergamot, lavender and vetiver). The more comfortable and experienced you get with blending essential oils; the more oils you can add to your blends.

For beginners, we recommend *starting with three oils*. One top note oil, then one middle note oil, and then one base note oil (for example: Bergamot, Lavender, and Vetiver). Once you become more comfortable and experienced, you can begin blending more essential oils.

Step 3 – Start to Blend Your Preferred Oils

You can **start blending oils** after you narrow down your choices. Base these choices on what the oils are being used for, and then narrow these choices down again based on notes and categories.

We recommend you **start with 10 drops of oil** total in order to test the new blend without wasting too much product. It's possible you may not like it later.

Note: work with undiluted essential oils at this stage. You are not yet using them with carrier oils. That is something that will come later. The "Dilution" chapter of this book can assist you with this.

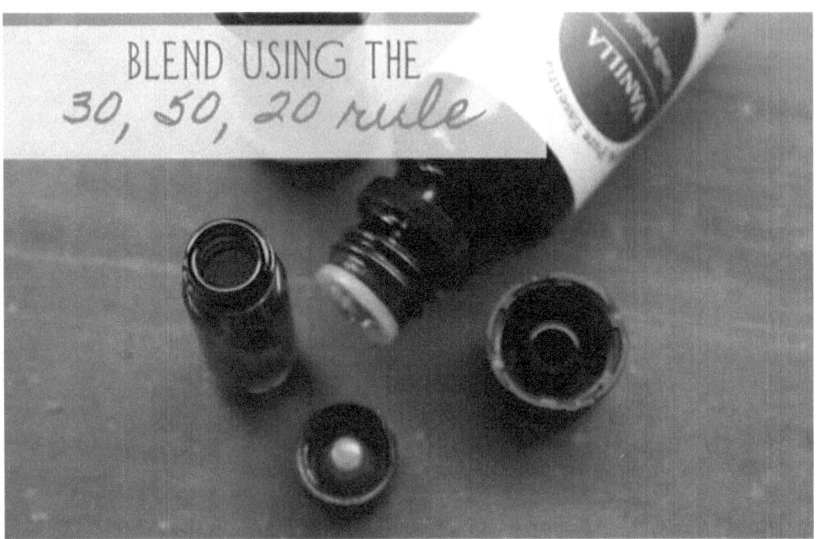

A commonly applied rule when it comes to producing essential oil blends is the *30, 50, 20 rule*.

- Use 30% of the *top note oil*.
- Use 50% of the *middle note oil*.
- Use 20% of the *base note oil*.

This formula is based on how quickly each oil will evaporate. When you apply your new blend, you will smell all the oils at the same time. As time passes, the top note will evaporate first. This means the blended aromas of the middle and base notes remain. As more time passes, the middle note evaporates and leaves only the base note.

Step 4 – Allow Your New Blend to Rest

Now that your oils are blended, set the blend aside to let it rest at least 24-48 hours. This will allow the constituents and chemicals for each essential oil to meld together, truly creating a proper blend among the three notes.

Step 5 – Test the New Blend

If you have reached this point, your blend has finished its resting period.

Now you can smell it to see how the oils have layered and if they complement each other.

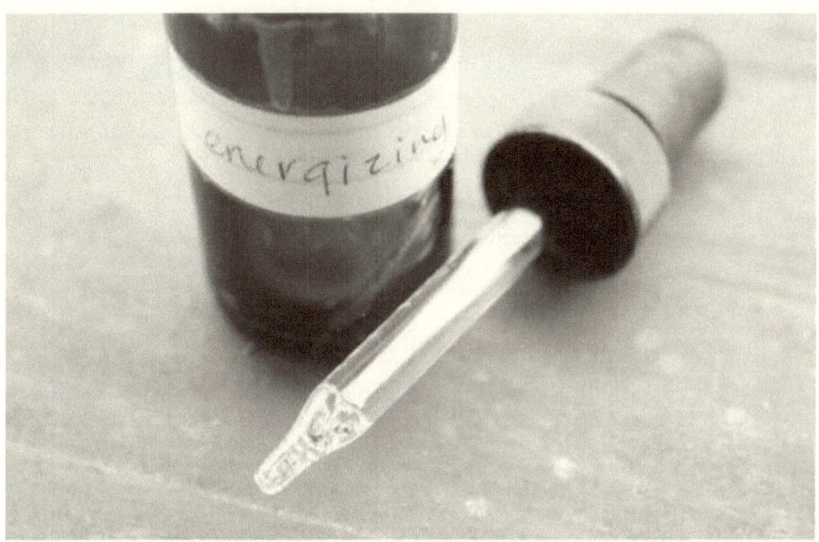

Once you have got the blend right, you can make up more of the oil, allow it to rest, and then bottle it up to use as necessary. Mastered that? You could try using a carrier oil to dilute your blend. There you have it, your very own essential oil blend!

8 Tested Blending Tips

1. Control how much oil you use, and ultimately how much you waste, by starting out with a small number of drops, no more than 25, when creating new blends.

2. Use essential oils *only* when you start creating blends. Wait until you include carrier oils so as not to waste them.

3. Keep a notebook of everything you do, because when the creative juices are flowing, you might forget exactly what was used or combined.

4. Perfume sample bottles are great for storage. They're inexpensive and easily found to purchase.

5. Make it a point to clearly label new blends. It isn't necessary to write down every detail, but you need some way to decipher what you've created.

6. It is important to use the *30, 50, 20 rule* when you first start blending.

7. Some oils are stronger than others. Unless your goal is for specific oils to dominate a new blend, it is best to do some research on what you're using. The internet is filled with online forums and resources that you can use to communicate with others.

8. After you finish a new blend, let it rest for 24-48 hours before making a decision about whether you love or hate it. The ingredients need time to adjust to one another.

HINTS FOR STORING ESSENTIAL OILS

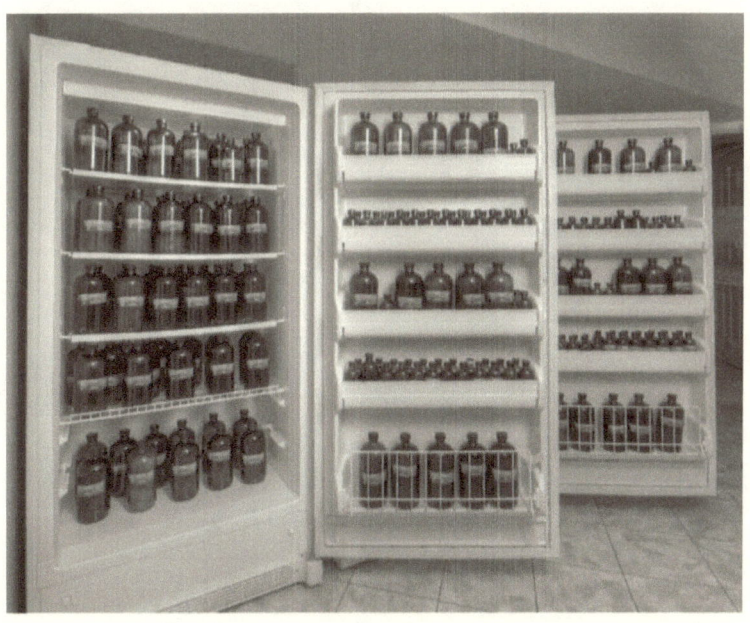

The way you look after your essential oils *will* affect their shelf life, so it's important to follow the correct procedure to save yourself time, money, and effort. Here is a great *'Do's and Don'ts'* guide:

1. *Don't* expose your essential oils to extreme or rapid changes in temperature.
2. *Do* keep your essential oils packaged in dark, colored glass because it filters out the sun's UV rays.
3. *Do* store your essential oils in a dark, cool place.

4. *Do* use the refrigerator to store your essential oils if you have the space.

5. *Don't* let your carrier oils get too warm as this will compromise the quality of the essential oils.

6. *Do* consider using an aromatherapy box if you don't have the room in your refrigerator. These are specifically designed to keep your essential oils at the desired temperature.

7. *Do* replace the cap of your essential oil bottles immediately after you have finished using them. They are prone to evaporating, and you don't want to risk losing them in this way.

8. *Don't* ever leave your essential oils near naked flame as they are highly flammable materials.

9. *Don't* ever decant your essential oils into plastic bottles as they will likely melt through it.

THE MOST COMMON APPLICATION TECHNIQUES

So now that we've looked at buying, diluting, and storing essential oils, it's time to talk about **proper application**. Getting this right is very important as it can help or hinder your recovery. There are **four** main application techniques: *aromatically, topically, internally, or externally*, all of which we are going to examine in detail through this chapter.

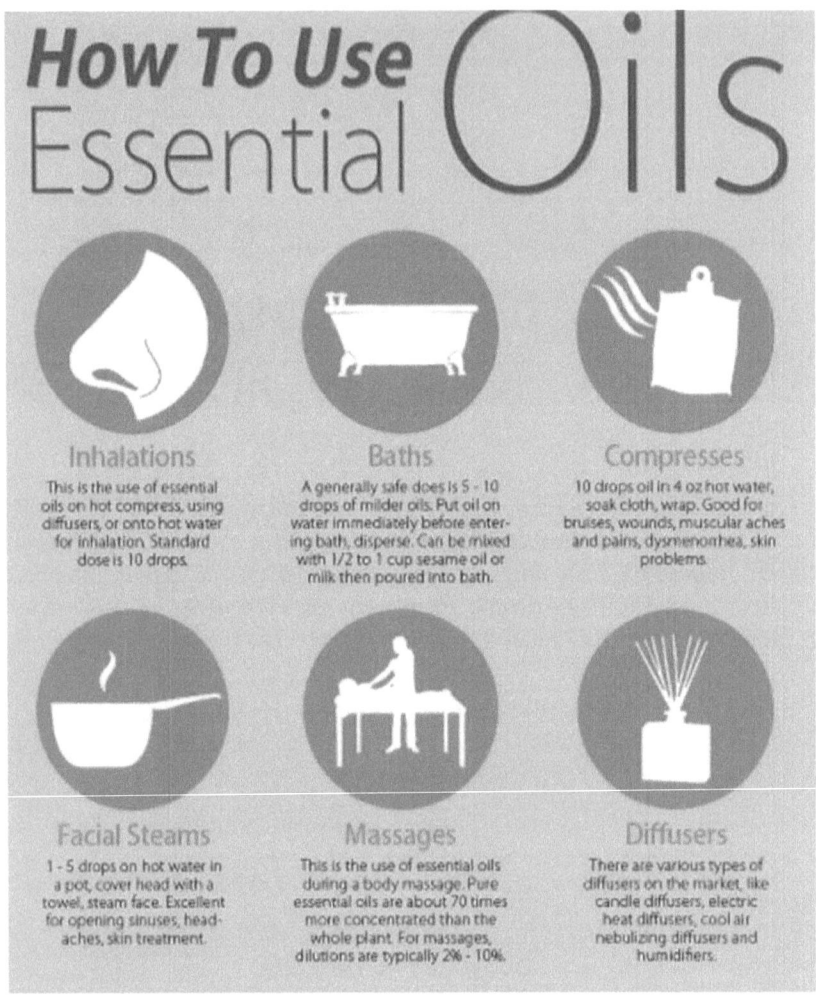

How To Use Essential Oils

Inhalations
This is the use of essential oils on hot compress, using diffusers, or onto hot water for inhalation. Standard dose is 10 drops.

Baths
A generally safe does is 5 - 10 drops of milder oils. Put oil on water immediately before entering bath, disperse. Can be mixed with 1/2 to 1 cup sesame oil or milk then poured into bath.

Compresses
10 drops oil in 4 oz hot water, soak cloth, wrap. Good for bruises, wounds, muscular aches and pains, dysmenorrhea, skin problems.

Facial Steams
1 - 5 drops on hot water in a pot, cover head with a towel, steam face. Excellent for opening sinuses, headaches, skin treatment.

Massages
This is the use of essential oils during a body massage. Pure essential oils are about 70 times more concentrated than the whole plant. For massages, dilutions are typically 2% - 10%.

Diffusers
There are various types of diffusers on the market, like candle diffusers, electric heat diffusers, cool air nebulizing diffusers and humidifiers.

Below is a guide to using essential oils correctly.

Aromatic

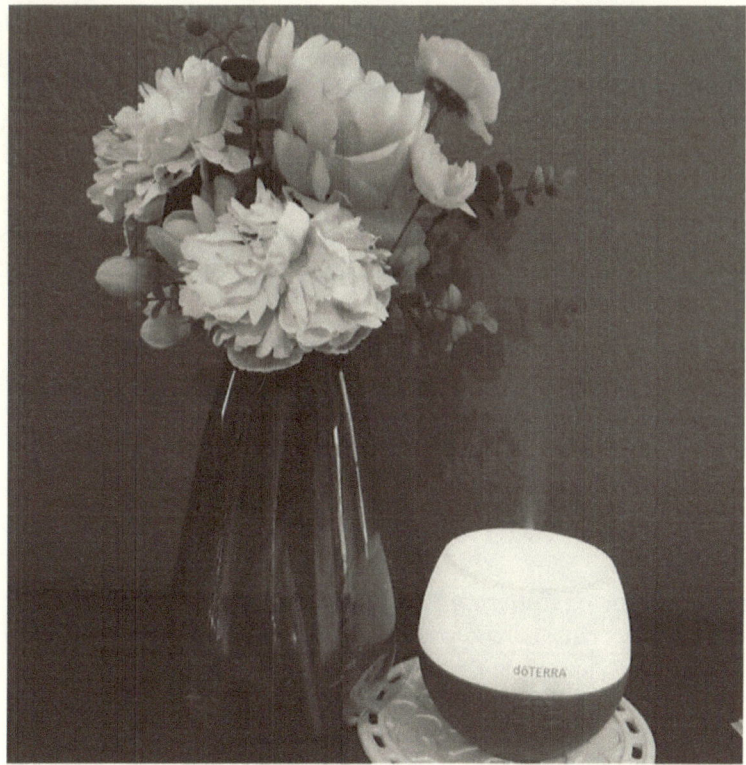

Aromatic is the most popular application for essential oils. This is because the positive properties of essential oils can be *inhaled* and then absorbed into your bloodstream. This method of application has several benefits.

- Nurtures your respiratory system.

- Offers a positive effect on your mood, tension, hormonal system, etc.

- Protects against airborne pollutants and enhances quality of indoor air.

- Boosts immune system response and improves well-being once an oil's effective compounds enter your bloodstream.

The methods for this type of application are:

- **Diffusers:** Diffusers will use cool to room temperature air, even ultrasonic vibrations, to send essential oils into the air. This helps oil molecules stay in the air longer and won't impact the oil's structure with heat, which may diminish its quality.

- **Inhalation (Direct and Indirect):** *Direct inhalation* works by holding the oil's bottle a couple inches from the nose, then breathing in or by rubbing a drop between your hands and cupping them over your nose and mouth. *Indirect inhalation* works by dropping essential oil onto a square of fabric, cotton ball, pillow case, or handkerchief and then breathing in the aroma from this oiled source.

- **Vapor/Steam Tent:** Heat (not to boil) a pot of water, then add 1-3 drops of your preferred oil. Drape a towel over your head as you lean over the steam and inhale.

- **Humidifier:** Humidifiers work similarly to a diffuser, where cool-air humidifiers work best. Note: essential oils may damage the plastic components over time; it's best to select one made specifically for essential oils.

- **Fan or Vent:** Working in a similar fashion to diffusers and indirect inhalation, add your preferred oil to a cloth and set it in a vent or on a fan.

- **Perfume or Cologne:** Add 1 drop of your preferred oil or oil blend to your wrists, behind your ears, or add 12 drops to 3 tsp. of distilled water or alcohol. Spritz this mix on your body or clothing. A mixture like this smells fresh and is healthier for your body compared to chemical-based colognes or perfumes.

- **Room Deodorizer:** Use essential oils in your room deodorizing efforts rather than harsh chemicals that only cover up odors. Make a blend that includes up to 40 drops of your favorite essential oil and equal parts alcohol (vodka works) and distilled water. Pour this mix into a decorative glass, jar, or vase and include kebob skewers (best if made from bamboo) long enough to stand up out of the top of the container. The bamboo soaks up the mixture, and the skewers act as a diffuser. If you prefer, create the same mixture and pour into a spray bottle for a more versatile and mobile application of the blend.

Note: when using essential oils aromatically, it's important to be aware of your body, your allergies and to take note of how you respond after you start to use the oils. Aromatic application is a potent use of essential oils, and using too much too often can overwhelm your senses or cause a reaction if you don't realize how sensitive you are to oils.

Topically

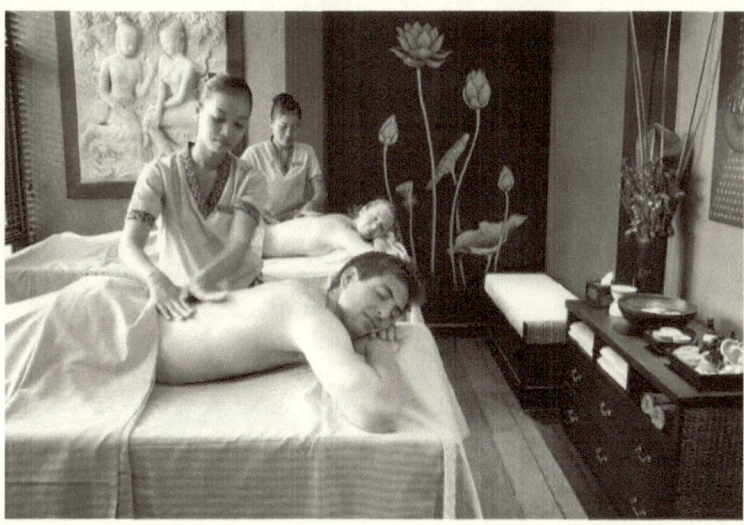

Mastering the topical use of essential oils can be a delicate, but fairly simple process. Please remember that *how* essential oils are used topically will vary from one oil to the next. Some oils will come with precautions, explaining how to dilute or how often an oil can be used. However, even those that don't come with precautions could affect some sensitive skin types, causing itchiness or a rash when not used carefully.

Before you use any oils topically, **know your skin type**. If you have sensitive skin, always dilute regardless of the oil you choose. Not sure? Perform a patch test on a spot along your inner arm. Always use *one oil at a time* and start with one diluted drop. If the undiluted oil is considered safe for use in most people, and the diluted drop produced no reaction, then try one undiluted drop. This way, you know exactly what you had a reaction to if there is any itchiness or other irritation.

It never hurts to dilute! Doing so won't decrease the oil's effectiveness and could help increase absorption because it prevents evaporation. As mentioned above, diluting will also decrease the likelihood of a negative skin reaction; without a solid reason not to, it's always a good idea to dilute.

- *Pure (or Neat) – Oils generally safe to use undiluted:* Generally, this means the oil can be applied directly to the skin without a carrier oil. It's always a good idea to patch test your skin, though, or follow the provided sensitivity guidelines when you know your skin is sensitive. Just remember, dilution never hurts and may help, if only by preventing skin irritation.

- ***Sensitive – Oils to be used with moderate dilution:*** Although some can apply oils directly to their skin without diluting, people with sensitive skin, especially children and the elderly, should always do a patch test or dilute before use. Follow the common guideline of mixing 1 drop of essential oil to 1-4 oz. of your preferred carrier oil or try 1 drop essential oil to every 3 drops of your preferred carrier oil.

- ***Dilute – Oils generally safe to use with heavier dilution:*** It's important to dilute **these very potent oils** at a ratio of *at least* 1:3, or possibly more, depending on a person's age and skin sensitivity. These oils could cause irritation when applied directly to any skin type. Consult your naturopathic doctor before use when you're pregnant or nursing. We recommend avoiding use for children; although, using high dilution rates with some oils could be acceptable in small amounts over limited periods of time.

There are other **topical precautions to remember**:

- *Citrus oils* may cause sensitivity to sunlight. Within 12 hours of topical application, we recommended avoiding going out in direct sunlight. For example, Bergamot has been known to cause sensitivity for almost 3 days. It would be best to apply these later in the day or to areas of the body that won't see direct sun exposure. Avoid topical use of citrus oils altogether when the above precautions can't be met.

- If you have sensitive skin or are prone to skin reactions, always use high dilution rates for the oils before use, then graduate to a lighter dilution if the oil is commonly recognized as one that can be used pure or "neat."

- Someone can develop a reaction to an oil after excessive use over the same area of the body, even if they don't think of their skin as sensitive. Combat this by alternating where you apply the oils *and* the oils you're using, remembering to dilute. It's possible you aren't aware of a sensitivity you have, which is why some experts will tell you to *always* dilute.

- Consider "layering" oils rather than blending them. This means that when using more than one topical oil, apply one, wait up to 30 minutes, then apply the second over it. Blending essential oils is an art and a science. This is why it may be safer using blends that a company has created.

The popular methods of topical essential oil applications are as follows:

- *Massage:* This is one of the most enjoyable topical uses of essential oils. Massaging essential oils into strained tissues, joints, and muscles is beneficial and relaxing. Avoid using a heavy hand or applying too much pressure while moving across sensitive areas. When massaging, make motions toward the heart while working on someone's arms and legs.

- *Directly to Area(s) of Concern:* This is the process of manually applying essential oils directly to the parts of the body that are experiencing pain, weakness, or strain (diluted when necessary). Areas of concern can also include the body's energy centers.

Directly to the Reflex Points: Learning how to apply essential oils in this way is supported by using visual guides explaining reflexology and which reflex points should be massaged considering the area of the body that is strained, weak, or in pain. The feet, hands, and ears are common reflex points, which affect different areas of the body via the nervous system. This is probably the most effective and gentlest application of essential oils, especially for sensitive skin, and for children or the elderly. You need to dilute as needed or directed because applying oils in this way can put them into the bloodstream quickly. For example, auricular therapy focuses on stimulating the small reflex points around the ears specifically.

Foot Reflexology Chart

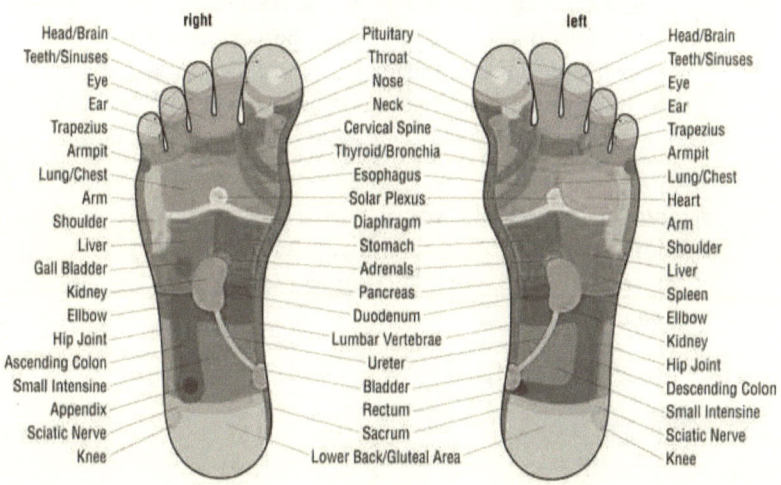

Hand Reflexology Chart

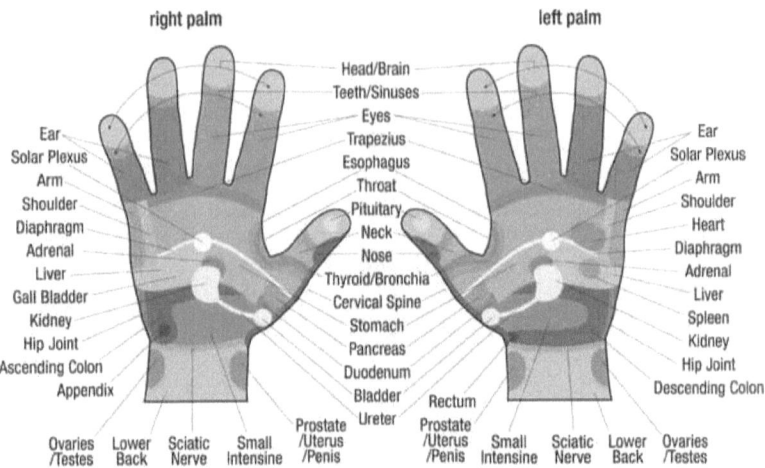

- *Auricular Therapy:* Similar to acupuncture, acupressure, or reflexology, auricular therapy stimulates small reflex points on and around the ears by massaging the essential oil into the area. (Try some Lavender to help calm an upset child.)

- *Use a Cold or Hot Compress:* A cold or hot compress consists of soaking a cloth or towel in cool water or wrapping a cloth or towel around a hot water bottle. Using either one of these with directly applied drops of your preferred essential oil can bring relief and relaxation to any area of concern.

- *Taking a Bath or Foot Bath:* Add several drops of your preferred essential oil to bathwater, bath salts, or a foot bath for soaking. If you're applying oils like this, it would be a good idea to mix them with carrier oils to disperse the oils and protect your body from collecting multiple drops all in one area – one that could be very sensitive!

- *Practicing Personal Care:* Essential oils can be used as a natural deodorant, added to lotion and moisturizers to relieve everything from irritated skin to fine lines, or as part of an antiaging skin-care regimen.

Internally

It is important to note that **not every essential oil should be consumed**, and each person should approach internal use with caution. Even though the *FDA* collected a list of essential oils that are "Generally Recognized as Safe" to consume, precaution is still needed. It is strongly advised to work with a health professional, an aromatherapist, before taking essential oils internally.

Applying essential oils internally requires more safety, more knowledge than other applications. These natural extracts are potent, and they can have a major impact – triggering allergic reactions being the smallest. The amounts you ultimately use won't be fatal, but they can be toxic to those who are already sensitive: children, the elderly, and pregnant or nursing women. Always check with a naturopathic doctor or other medicinal professional before use, read labels carefully, shop from trusted vendors, and keep your oils, especially ones with familiar food scents, away from child-accessible spaces.

Some of the most recognized precautions are:

- *Be conservative:* Think in terms of the patch test. Start with one drop of the oil you want to use, see what effects it generates, then graduate to larger amounts slowly.

- *Start with small amounts more frequently:* Similar to above, to protect your liver you want to start small – using one drop every 45 minutes, or so, for instance – and not use 5 drops in one dosage. Graduate up to this amount slowly.

- *Consider the circumstances:* Think about the area of concern and determine if internal use is the best application to treat the problem. Because of the potential for negative effects, save internal application for when it is really needed.

- *Know your limits:* Most herbalists will warn against consuming more than 25 drops of oils in one day (especially citrus oils). Aim for consuming around 10 drops per day, after gaining thorough knowledge of how your body responds, and just remember: you don't have to use an oil if you don't really *need* it daily.

- *Know your oils:* Some oils, for example Thyme, Oregano, and Cinnamon, have a high phenol concentration that can accumulate in your liver. This is why it is always important to use oils with care. There are books, websites, and groups or experts online easily accessible enough for you to take some time and really get familiar with the oils you want to use.

- *It never hurts to dilute:* There are plenty of edible carrier oils available, Olive, Jojoba, Coconut, Sweet Almond, and Apricot Kernel oils, to name a few, that there is no reason to avoid diluting before internal application – even when you use capsules to consume your oils.

- *Know your sensitivities:* You'll see this a lot in this book, but women who are pregnant or nursing, children and the elderly, and people with a major health concern, such as liver issues or an otherwise compromised immune system, might be safer simply avoiding the internal use of most oils. Speak with an herbalist or trusted medicinal/herbal professional before every use.

If you are ready to use an oil internally, these are suggestions for **applying essential oils internally**:

- *In food and beverages:* Several oils are added to meals, baked goods, or beverages. If you would add the herbs to food or as a flavor to water, you can use the essential oils (a single drop or less) in the same way: Oregano, Thyme, Basil, Lemon, or Peppermint are some great examples. Of course, start with a small number of drops at first. When it comes to beverages, some great "carrier" drinks are water and almond or rice milk. Be sure to mix well, though, because **oil and water will not mix**. The oil will visibly float toward the top, forcing you to consume too much at once.

- *As a supplement:* Consider the multivitamins you buy at the store and take daily. Much like that, you can use essential oils internally by adding them to a substance like honey or blending them and inserting them into an empty capsule. Boost your immunity, energy, or digestion with a pre-made blend from an herbalist or well-trusted vendor.

Suppository or enema: Insertion into a body orifice, vaginal or rectal, is a far more advanced internal application technique than any we've discussed so far. Discovering sensitivity to oils this way is not a comfortable experience. Ease into this kind of internal application by diluting the oil of choice in a soothing carrier oil before adding to warm bathwater, then soak up to 20 minutes.

Externally

Here are a few extra ideas for **using essential oils around the home**:

- Use these essential oils around the house for:
    - Melaleuca: add to sink before washing dishes
    - Lemon: stain remover, air freshener
    - Arborvitae or Peppermint: repel crawling insects
    - Lemongrass and Eucalyptus: repel mosquitoes
    - Lime: removes sticky residues such as gum, tape, or stickers
- Give laundry day a boost by adding a few drops of oils, diluted with water, to a spray bottle and spritzing clothes before they go on the line or into the dryer. Or, you can add them, undiluted, directly to the barrel of the washing machine before you start your first load.
- Look for oils that have antifungal or antiviral properties. Include them with blends to use as household cleaners, carpet powders and deodorizers, or furniture polish.
- Improve the aroma of craft paint and supplies, paint for the house, or children's clay or dough by adding essential oils to the mix. You could use as much as an entire bottle of oils (for a gallon of paint, for instance) to as little as 2 drops (for the children's dough).

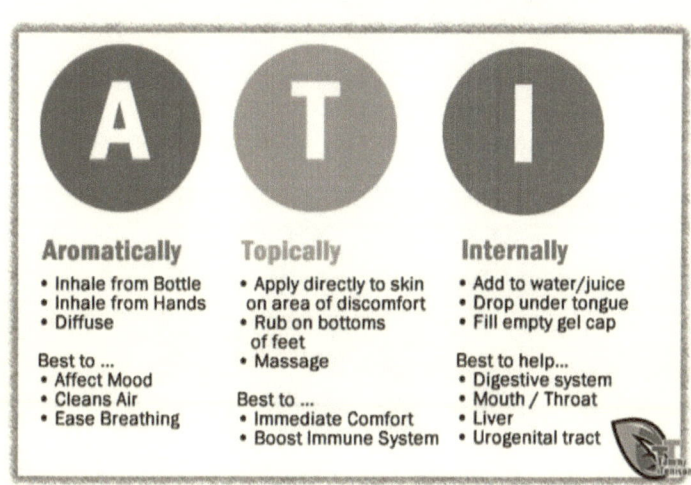

SAFETY TIPS FOR ESSENTIAL OIL USAGE

One of the most important things to think about when coming to essential oil use is safety.

Factors to consider toward essential oil safety:

- **Quality** – Before buying a single essential oil make sure you conduct thorough research on the vendor, know if the oil being sold is pure and authentic, and know what they are diluted with if you are buying them adulterated or in pre-made blends.

- **Composition** – Some compounds that appear naturally in essential oils, such as phenols and aldehydes, can cause adverse or allergic reactions. This is why it never hurts to dilute an essential oil before each use.

- **Application** – Each of the four application methods – internal, topical, diffused, or inhaled – has its own safety precautions that need to be understood before each use.

- **Dosage** – Be sure to follow blend recipes carefully, look at the ingredients of each pre-made blend you use, and double-check suggested dosages for each application method, clearly considering the area of concern first. When in doubt, or if you know you have sensitivities or sensitive skin, don't be afraid to dilute with water or a carrier oil of your choice before each use.

- **Area of concern** – Skin that is inflamed, damaged, or diseased can be more susceptible to essential oils because it is more permeable. Applying undiluted oils to skin in this condition makes negative dermal reactions more likely. When in doubt, dilute or drop the dosage for skin extra sensitive due to injury, damage, or disease.

Possible Dermal Reactions

Use of essential oils may cause skin, or dermal, reactions such as sensitization, irritation, and photosensitization.

Dermal irritant – Produces immediate effects on your skin. This may appear as redness, blotchiness, or pain. Dilution or dosage of the essential oil that was applied will directly impact severity of the dermal irritation. The chart below gives some examples of these:

Essential Oil	Latin Name
Bay	*Pimento racemosa*
Cinnamon bark or leaf	*Cinnamomum zeylanicum**
Clove bud	*Syzygium aromaticum*
Citronella	*Cymbopogon nardus*
Cumin	*Cuminum cyminum*
Lemongrass	*Cymbopogon citratus*
Lemon verbena	*Lippia citriodora*
Oregano	*Origanum vulgare*
Tagetes	*Tagetes minuta*
Thyme ct. thymol	*Thymus vulgaris*

*bark is more irritating than leaf

Dermal sensitization – Occurs upon initial skin exposure, a kind of allergic reaction similar to the irritation described above, but any visible effect is slight. It is after subsequent exposure to the same, or a similar, material when the immune system kicks in and produces a severe inflammatory response.

Once that response occurs, the individual will most likely remain sensitive to that specific essential oil for many years if not the rest of their life. This is why it is important to dilute oils before use and only use oils when needed, not just because you have them.

Essential Oil	Latin Name
Cassia	*Cinnamomum cassia*
Cinnamon bark	*Cinnamomum zeylanicum*
Peru balsam	*Myroxylon pereirae*
Verbena absolute	*Lippia citriodora*
Tea absolute	*Camellia sinensis*
Turpentine oil	*Pinus spp.*
Backhousia	*Backhousia citriodora*
Inula	*Inula graveolens*
Oxidized oils from Pinaceae family (e.g., Pinus and Cupressus species) and Rutaceae family (e.g., citrus oils)	

Photosensitization – Also known as phototoxicity, this reaction occurs when an essential oil increases the skin's sensitivity to direct sunlight. Photosensitization may present as burning or changes to skin pigmentation, to as extreme as weeping burns. Avoid the use of essential oils with this property prior to spending any extended amount of time in direct sunlight or a tanning booth. We recommend waiting at least 24 hours after applying known photosensitizing essential oils.

The following essential oils are considered as photo sensitizers:

Essential Oil	Latin Name
Angelica root	*Angelica archangelica*
Bergamot	*Citrus bergamia*
Cumin	*Cuminum cyminum*
Distilled or expressed grapefruit (low risk)	*Citrus paradisi*

Expressed lemon	*Citrus limon*
Expressed lime	*Citrus medica*
Orange, bitter (expressed)	*Citrus aurantium*
Rue	*Ruta graveolens*

The table below includes a list of non-phototoxic citrus oils:

Essential Oil	Latin Name
Bergamot: Bergapteneless (FCF: Furanocoumarin Free)	*Citrus bergamia*
Distilled lemon	*Citrus limon*
Distilled lime	*Citrus medica*
Mandarin – Tangerine	*Citrus reticulata*
Sweet orange	*Citrus sinensis*
Expressed tangerine	*Citrus reticulata*
Yuzu oil (expressed or distilled)	*Citrus juno*

Idiosyncratic sensitization – Idiosyncratic sensitization can also present as skin irritation. This is an unusual response to an essential oil that is otherwise commonly used. These responses are unpredictable and rarely occur, but be on the lookout for them when using essential oils.

Mucous membrane irritant – Produces a drying or heating effect on the reproductive organs, nose, eyes, or mouth. We recommend not using mucous membrane-irritating oils without the use of a moisturizing or soothing carrier oil. These oils can have the strongest effect when used in oil blends that go in the bath. Avoid this by always using a carrier oil, waiting to add the oils until after the water has been added to the bathtub, and completely avoiding use of Lemongrass, Cinnamon Bark, Bay, Thyme ct. thymol, and Clove.

Essential Oil	Latin Name
Bay	*Pimento racemosa*
Caraway	*Carum carvi*
Cinnamon bark or leaf	*Cinnamomum zeylanicum*
Clove bud or leaf	*Syzygium aromaticum*
Lemongrass	*Cymbopogon citratus*
Peppermint	*Mentha x piperita*
Thyme ct. thymol	*Thymus vulgaris*

Other Safety Considerations

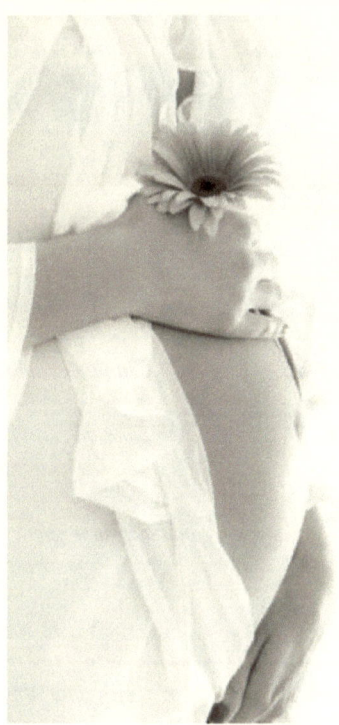

Pregnancy – As it has been stated previously, pregnant women are extra sensitive to many essential oils and are told to avoid most altogether. The main concern is that essential oil compounds could pass through the placenta and negatively affect the fetus. Risk to the fetus is directly related to the concentration of the toxic compounds in the essential oil.

These **essential oils appear safe for pregnant women:** Rosewood, Cardamom, Neroli, Rose, Sandalwood, Chamomile (after asking your trusted herbal professional), Petitgrain, Frankincense, Patchouli, and Geranium. Test and use caution with other nontoxic oils; it would be safer to avoid internal or undiluted application of any oil.

The following table outlines **the essential oils you should avoid while pregnant, giving birth, and breastfeeding.**

Essential Oil	Latin Name
Aniseed	*Pimpinella anisum*
Angelica	*Angelica arhangelica*
Basil ct. estragole	*Ocimum basilicum*
Birch	*Betula lenta*
Black Pepper	*Piper nigrum*
Camphor	*Cinnamomum camphora*
Cinnamon	*Cinnamomum verum, Cinnamomum zeylanicum*
Chamomile	*Chamaemelum nobile, Chamaemelum matricaria*
Clary Sage	*Salvia sclarea*
Clove	*Syzygium aromaticum*
Fennel	*Foeniculum vulgare*
Fir	*Abies alba, abies balsamea, abies grandis*
Ginger	*Zingiber officinale*
Horseradish	*Armoracia lapathifolia gilib*
Hyssop	*Hyssopus officinalis*
Jasmine	*Jasminum officinalis*
Juniper	*Juniperus Communis*
Marjoram	*Origanum majorana*
Mugwort	*Artemisia vulgaris*
Mustard	*Brassica nigra, Brassica hirta*

Myrrh	*Commiphora myrrha*
Nutmeg	*Myristica fragrans*
Oregano	*Origanum vulgare*
Parsley seed or leaf	*Petroselinum sativum*
Pennyroyal	*Mentha pulegium*
Peppermint	*Mentha x Piperita*
Rosemary	*Rosmarinus officinalis*
Sage	*Salvia officinalis*
Tansy	*Tanacetum vulgare*
Tarragon	*Artemisia dracunculus*
Thuja	*Thuja occidentalis*
Thyme	*Thymus vulgaris*
Wintergreen	*Gaultheria procumbens*
Wormwood	*Artemisia absinthium*

Eye safety – When using essential oils, you must be careful with your eyes. The following tips are considered the most important:

- Do not apply undiluted oils to your eyes. They are not typically used to alleviate eye trauma.
- Products used to treat eye diseases or injuries are considered medicine, regulated by drug legislation. No medical evidence exists to prove that applying essential oils to eye trauma will be beneficial.
- Notable exception: Tea Tree oil that has been diluted, used alongside an anesthetic eyedrop, can kill eyelash mites.

General Safety Precautions

1. Store essential oils away from child- and pet-accessible spaces.

2. Wait at least 24 hours before going into direct sunlight or a tanning booth after applying oils that have photosensitizing properties.

3. Alternate use of essential oils; rotate oils in the same family and treatment areas on your body.

4. Research every essential oil before you use it; know the safety precautions, take them.

5. Remember: it never hurts to dilute.

6. Perform a patch test before every use.

7. Use caution when trying to conceive, when pregnant or breastfeeding.

8. Do not use essential oils in your eyes.

9. Keep essential oils away from open flames, including gas cookers and cigarettes.

10. Give yourself proper ventilation when blending, using, or treating with essential oils.

11. Get trained in the safety procedures for internal application of essential oils.

Safety Measures

- Essential oil in your eyes: Use a cloth and a fixed oil, like Sesame or Olive, then swipe the cloth across the closed lid. Also try flushing with cool water.

- Essential oil causes skin irritation or sensitization: Apply fixed oil, like vegetable, or a soothing cream to affected area. Stop using that product.

- Essential oil is consumed by a child: Do not try to get the child to vomit; try getting them to drink 2% or whole milk. Find and keep the essential oil bottle for accurate identification. Check the telephone directory, call local poison control department for further direction.

WHY ESSENTIAL OILS?

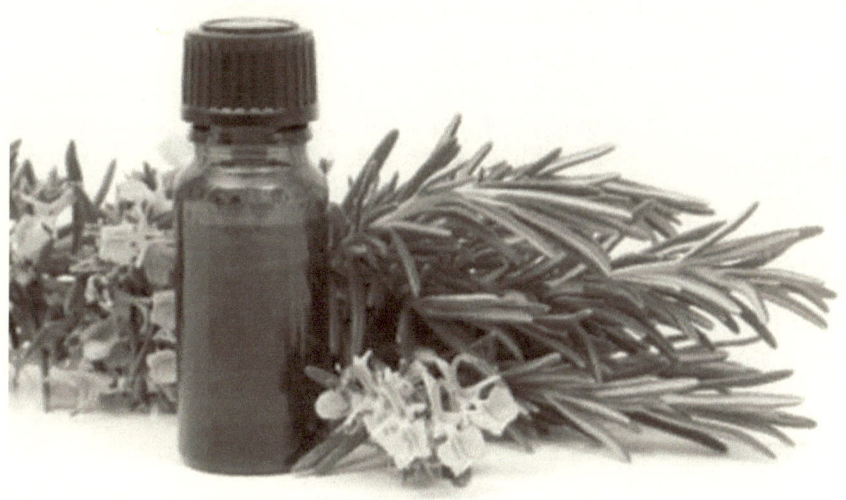

So now that we've looked at the reasons people are turning away from tradi-tional medication for treating their ailments, it's time to examine *why* essential oils are not only a better option, but the most effective way to treat the most common ailments.

Benefits

According to most sources, the Top Benefits for choosing essential oils are:

- They are **easy** (and fun) to use, and work!
- They are **nontoxic** to our body, our kids, and our pets (only if used correctly). Not all oils are safe for children, and be careful when using essential oils with cats.
- They are good for the planet and our **environment**.
- They support the improvement of physical and emotional **well-being**.
- They improve the **quality** of our lives.
- They give us an alternative healing solution.
- They have more **benefits** than side effects.

There are many different types of traditional medication that can have a very negative impact on your health, with very little help. Another issue long-term users of medication often come across is **tolerance**. They become so *used* to their medication, that it no longer works as effectively. This is when we need to start looking at something new.

What you might not know about essential oils is that they can actually heal you at a cellular level. This means the level of help that they can give you when it comes to your ailments is phenomenal.

The
TOP FIVE
Benefits Of
Essential Oils

Less Irritating

Essential oils are less irritating to the skin and better for people with allergies than products made with synthetic fragrances.

Pure

The fragrances you enjoy from essential oils are pure and of the highest quality.

Atmosphere Creating

Essential oils can be used to create different moods and atmospheres in your everyday environment. Since they are completely natural, essential oils combine better with each other and create more graceful and sophisticated combinations than artificial fragrances.

Holistic Healing

A candle made with lavender and lemon essential oils will bring balance, peace, and cheerfulness. A diffuser of lime and mint essential oils encourages mental clarity and alertness.

Longer Lasting

While the fragrance of a lotion made with synthetic lavender may deteriorate within six months to a year, a lotion made with natural essential oils will last for several years.

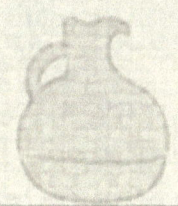

Side Effects Of Essential Oils

Now, you may know that essential oils work differently to traditional medicine, but you might not know *why* or why they aren't included in the same field.

What we do know about essential oils comes from information that has been passed down through centuries of experimentation and private use. This is because essential oils are technically naturally occurring substances, which means they will never be regulated by patent laws. That makes a pharmaceutical company less likely to include essential oils in a manmade drug. So, mainstream healthcare practitioners are even less likely to even suggest essential oils as a medicinal or therapeutic alternative. Without a drug company's interest based on patents, money won't get invested to study essential oils. This **greatly** limits our scientific knowledge of essential oils.

Despite the fact that these oils are wholly natural, they still carry **a risk of side effects**. Even though the side effects of essential oils are nothing compared to what you will get from traditional medicine, there are some things to look out for. After all, it's better to be safe than sorry!

The following are rare side effects to look out for:

- **Skin Discoloration** – This is caused by photosensitizing essential oils, such as Cumin, Lemon, Bergamot, and Lime. Remember to wait 24 hours before you spend time in direct sunlight or lay in a tanning booth. Skin irritation can be as minor as discoloration or as bad as oozing burns.

- **Pregnancy Complications** – To avoid complication for pregnant and breastfeeding women, essential oils should always be heavily diluted or avoided completely. There are safe carrier oils, such as Sweet Almond or Coconut oil. On the other hand, Spike Lavender and Rosemary should always be avoided. It would be most safe to only use products designated for pregnant women. Do some research online with The National Association for Holistic Aromatherapy to see what they recommend when it comes to essential oils and oil blends.

- **Skin Irritation** – To avoid serious skin irritation always perform a patch test before using any essential oils on your skin. When using oils such as Bay, Citronella, Lemongrass, or Cinnamon, make sure it is diluted in a soothing carrier oil. Never assume any essential oil is safe for direct topical application.

- **Small Pets Are Sensitive** – Do not use essential oils directly on small pets. Contact your veterinarian and ask specific questions before using essential oil products on your pet.

- **Danger to Pre-existing Illnesses** – People with pre-existing conditions may want to avoid use of essential oils; these people are even more sensitive to side effects. When treating others, ask specific questions to a trained aromatherapist, who has spent more than 200 hours taking chemistry classes and studying drug interactions.

- **Swallowing May Lead to Death or Illness** – Only take oils orally after you have complete knowledge and understanding of the oil's effects. There are fatal oils out there, like Wintergreen and Pennyroyal; others are so toxic they can lead to miscarriage. Even oils that have spent too much time on the shelf can become very irritating. Only apply internally if you're using oils with the guidance of an herbal or medical professional.

These scenarios are very extreme but, considering that, you should always consult a health professional before taking any products. Remember that they are a medication and should be treated as such.

Essential Oils and Pharmaceuticals Compared

Essential Oils	Pharmaceuticals
Properties	Properties
1. Natural, wildcrafted or grown organically	1. Unnatural, synthetic chemically or genetically engineered
2. Hundreds of constituents, not all known	2. One or two active ingredients, all of which are known
3. Never two batches the same.	3. Every batch the same (Purity)
4. Not patentable (God made)	4. Patentable (man made)
Effects and Consequences	Effects and Consequences
5. Restores natural function	5. Inhibits natural function
6. No adverse interactions	6. Many adverse interactions
7. Antiviral	7. Usually not antiviral
8. Improves intercellular communication	8. Disrupts intercellular communication
9. Corrects and restores proper cellular memory (DNA)	9. Garbles and confuses cellular memory (DNA)
10. Cleanses receptor sites	10. Blocks receptor sites
11. Builds the immune system	11. Depresses immune system
12. Emotionally balancing	12. Emotionally unbalancing
13. Side effects beneficial	13. Side effects harmful
14. Leads toward independence and wellness	14. Leads toward dependence and chronic disease
Philosophy/Paradigm	Philosophy/Paradigm
15. Assumes wellness as natural state, invulnerable to illness	15. Assumes natural state prone and vulnerable to illness
16. Assumes body and mind capable of self-healing	16. Assumes body and mind need external assistance to heal
17. Integrated wholistically, body, mind, and soul as a unit	17. Fragmented, treats body parts, mind and emotions separate
18. Build natural defenses and let body deal with disease	18. Supplant natural defenses and attack disease itself
19. Treats internally at level of cellular intelligence	19. Treats externally at level of gross symptoms
20. Theistic, historic roots in religion when healers were priests	20. Secular, historic roots in materialism motivated by money

ESSENTIAL OILS FOR COMMON AILMENTS

As previously stated, there are essential oils for pretty much everything! This chapter is going to look at how essential oils can help with a huge range of common ailments.

(15) essential oils
for every ailment

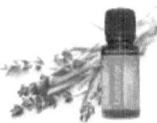

lavender
» calming & relaxing
» eases skin irritations
» supports skin healing

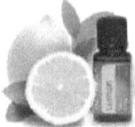

lemon
» aromatic cleanser
» internal detoxifier
» uplifts mood & energy

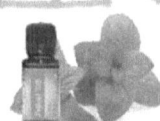

peppermint
» supports respiratory
function & oral health
» eases digestion & headaches

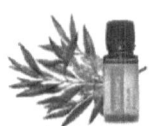

melaleuca
» cleanse & rejuvenate skin
» promotes healthy immune
function

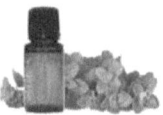

oregano
» supports digestion
» aids immune function
» powerful antioxidant

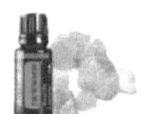

frankincense
» supports immune system
» uplifts mood
» aids in skin healing

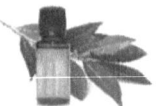

respiratory blend
» supports respiratory
health for clearer breathing
» aids in restful sleep

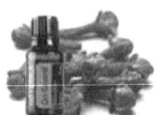

protective blend
» support healthy immune function
» non-toxic cleaner for the home
» purifies the air & environment

soothing blend
» soothes sore muscles
» comforts achey joints
» supports circulation

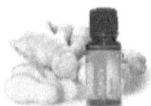

digestive blend
» aids digestion
» maintains healthy GI tract
» soothes stomach upset

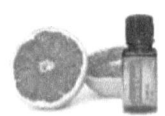

metabolic blend
» promotes healthy metabolism
» energizing & uplifting
» help manage cravings

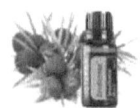

detox blend
» supports healthy detox
» aids in liver function
» purifies body systems

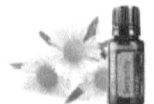

calming blend
» relaxes mind & body
» promotes restful sleep
» promotes sense of well-being

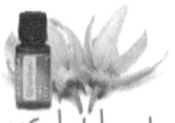

joyful blend
» mood-elevating effect
» revitalize mind & body
» energizing & refreshing

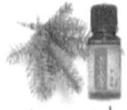

grounding blend
» warm, woody aroma
» promotes calm & well-being
» evokes tranquility & balance

These oils will all be examined in the next chapter – "Top Oils" – but here is a guide about the most popular oils for the most common ailments:

Uses of the Essential Oils

NAME	Suggested USES
Basil – *Ocium Basilicum*	Soothing, Energizing, Toning. Invigorates body and spirit. Relieves brain fatigue, nervousness, anxiety, depression, tension headaches, nervous insomnia, mental overwork, high stress working environment, tension related sexual problems.
Bergamot – *Citrus Bergamia*	Relaxes and refreshes and is good for confidence building. Good for stress and irritability, critical and exacting person with edgy and raw nerves.
Black Pepper – *Piper Nigrum*	Circulatory stimulant, warming and digestive. Excess mucous, head colds and flu. Warming before sports and cold hands and feet.
Chamomile	Sedative for calming and relief of pain. Nerves, headache, insomnia and menstrual disorders. Good for protecting dry skin.
Cedarwood – *Cedrus Atlantica*	Balancing and regenerating for nervous tension, anxiety, depression and tiredness, arthritis, chronic diarrhea, excessive discharges, for those prone to daydreams and fantasies.
Clary Sage B1 – *Salvia Sclarea*	Uplifts the spirit. Soothes, relaxes and warms and sedating, for depression, postnatal depression, frigidity, impotence, muscle relaxant, effective labor oil to strengthen contractions and for PMT, and menopause.
Cypress – *Cypresses Semipirverins*	Astringent to the circulatory system for varicose veins and broken capillaries, hemorrhoids, excessive discharges, nosebleeds, relieves heavy prolonged menstrual bleeding and menopause.

Eucalyptus – *Eucalyptus Globulus*	Powerful antiseptic, warming and drying, for tiredness, poor concentration, headaches, colds, flu, sinusitis, bronchitis, decongestant, rheumatism and arthritis, itching of insect bites, lack of direction in life.
Fennel – *Foeniculum Vulgare Dulce*	Moving, "unblocking oil", digestive stimulant, relieves flatulence, spastic colon, coughs, diuretic, detoxifying, cellulite, increases milk production, engorged breasts, helps express feelings.
Geranium – *Pelargonium Odorantissimum*	Balancing, regulating, for menopausal symptoms, hot flushes, restlessness, anxiety, panic attacks, anti-inflammatory, cystitis, dry eczema, for stuck, fearful people, low self-esteem.
Ginger – *Zingiber Officinale*	Warming, for colds, flu, fevers, headaches, nausea, immune stimulant, arthritis, rheumatism, muscle aches and pains, and for those frequently side-tracked.
Grapefruit – *Citrus Paradisi*	Cooling, refreshing, detoxifying, irritability, anger, overheating, constipation, cellulite, obesity, lymphatic cleansing, colds, flu hot fevers, for self-conscious, unhappy people, gives self-worth.
Jasmine B1 – *Jasminum Officinale*	Uplifting, promotes a state of relaxed awareness, anti-depressant, de-stresses, aphrodisiac, eases menstrual discomfort, labor pain, for time of trauma and grief, encourages acceptance.
Juniper berry – *Juniperus Communis*	Warming and stimulating, detoxifying, cystitis, boosts sluggish systems, fluid retention, obesity, cellulite, gout rheumatism and arthritis, eliminates uric acid, for people who fear rejection.
Lavender – *Lavandula Augustifolia*	Balancing, regulating, sedating, for irritability, depression, insomnia, hysteria, shock and nervous tension, headaches, neuralgia, shingles, sciatica, muscular pains, rheumatism, for sensitive people.

Lemon – *Citrus Limonum*	Refresher, anti-bacterial, sluggish circulation, varicose veins, broken capillaries, obesity, cellulite, detoxifying, immune stimulant, colds and flu, warts, wrinkles, greasy skin and hair.
Lemongrass – *Cymbopogon Citratus*	Refreshing, antiseptic, for sluggish digestion, colitis, enteritis, poor muscle tone, static tissues, pre-sport, aching, strained muscles post-sport, for people who feel like victims and are taken for granted.
Mandarin – *Citrus Reticulata*	Moving oil, for conditions where stagnation and putrefaction are present, suitable for children, gentle and calming, hyperactivity, stress and nervous insomnia, encourages peristalsis.
Neroli – *Citrus Auratium*	Calms, relaxes and uplifts the spirit and helps maintain confidence, anti-depressant, clears confusion, shock hysteria, heart palpitations, rejuvenates the skin, stretch marks, encourages the expression of emotions and heart feelings.

Below is a guide for **the most common ailments and use of essential oils** for those ailments.

COMMON AILMENT	ESSENTIAL OILS TO USE	HOW TO APPLY
Aches and Pain	Basil, Black Pepper, Chamomile, Cinnamon, Clove, Cypress, Ginger, Juniper, Lavender, Marjoram, Rosemary, Thyme, Ylang Ylang	Massage, Compress, Bath, Vaporization, Inhalation
Acid Reflux	Peppermint	Take in capsule or apply topically on stomach.
Acne	Basil, Bergamot, Cedarwood, Cypress, Geranium, Grapefruit, Lavender, Palmarosa, Rose, Tea Tree	Bath, or apply topically on location and massage.
ADD/ADHD	Lavender, Cedarwood, Vetiver	Diffuse or inhale directly, can be applied topically on the bottoms of feet.
Addictions	Bergamot	Can be diffused or applied topically over the liver.
Allergies	Lavender, Lemon, Peppermint, Eucalyptus	Can be infused or inhaled, applied topically on sinuses and bottoms of feet or taken in capsule.
Anger	Lavender	Can be infused or inhaled or applied over the heart and on bottoms of feet.
Anxiety	Lavender, Orange	Can be infused or inhaled or applied to the back of neck or temples.
Arthritis	Frankincense, Marjoram	Can be diffused or applied on location with a warm compress.

Asthma	Chamomile, Eucalyptus, Frankincense, Myrtle, Myrrh, Peppermint, Pine	Bath, Massage into chest, throat or back, Vaporization, Inhalation
Athlete's Foot	Lavender, Lemon, Myrrh, Tea Tree	Bath, Direct Application
Bacterial Infection	Tea Tree, Cinnamon, Peppermint	Can be diffused or applied on location or to liver area or bottoms of feet.
Bee Sting	Basil, Roman Chamomile	Apply topically on location. Place cool compress on it.
Bleeding	Helichrysum, Geranium	Apply topically on location.
Bronchitis	Eucalyptus, Thyme, Basil	Can be diffused or inhaled, applied topically to chest, sinuses, neck or feet.
Burns	Lavender, Geranium	Apply topically on location.
Chest Problems	Frankincense, Myrtle, Myrrh, Niaouli, Pine, Rosemary, Tea Tree, Thyme	Bath, Massage, Vaporization, Inhalation
Chilblains	Black Pepper, Cedarwood, Ginger, Juniper, Marjoram, Thyme	Massage, Bath, Compress
Colds and Flu	Basil, Black Pepper, Cinnamon, Eucalyptus, Ginger, Lavender, Lemon, Myrtle, Niaouli, Peppermint, Pine, Tea Tree, Thyme	Bath, Massage and apply to throat, temples, forehead and sinuses; diffuse, Inhale from water vapor.
Congestion	Eucalyptus, Peppermint	Apply to chest, neck and back or diffuse and inhale directly or from water vapor.

Constipation	Black Pepper, Clary Sage, Cypress, Eucalyptus, Peppermint, Rosemary	Bath, Massage – apply over the stomach; Compress
Corns	Clove	Apply topically on location.
Coughs	Tea Tree, Eucalyptus	Diffuse and inhale directly or apply topically on throat and chest.
Cramp	Chamomile, Lavender, Marjoram, Sandalwood, Vetiver	Bath, Massage, Compress
Cuts/Wounds	Helichrysum, Lavender, Tea Tree	Apply topically on location
Cystitis	Chamomile, Lavender, Tea Tree, Geranium, Pine, Sandalwood	Bath, Massage, Compress
Dandruff	Cedarwood, Lavender, Lemongrass, Sandalwood	Scalp massage, rinse
Depression	Frankincense, Lavender, Orange, Lemon	Diffuse or inhale directly, or apply topically to forehead; Massage or bath. Can also be taken internally 1-2 drops in capsule or water.
Diarrhea	Chamomile, Lavender, Rose, Neroli, Peppermint, Ginger, Geranium	Bath, Massage, Warm Compress. Apply topically to abdomen.
Earache	Basil, Tea Tree, Melrose, Helichrysum	Apply to surface of ear, behind ear, or swab around ear canal.
Eczema	Chamomile, Lavender, Myrrh, Sandalwood, Vetiver	Bath, Massage
Energy	Peppermint	Inhale directly or infuse; Massage, Bath.

Fever	Peppermint, Lemon, Eucalyptus, Clove	Swallow in capsule or apply topically to back or bottoms of feet or diffuse
Fleas	Citronella	Apply topically on location
Fluid Retention	Black Pepper, Cypress, Juniper	Bath, Massage
Fungal Infection	Tea Tree, Oregano, Thyme, Clove	Apply topically on location; use warm compress.
Gas/Flatulence	Peppermint, Ginger	Apply to stomach or feet
Hay Fever	Bergamot, Cedarwood, Chamomile, Eucalyptus, Geranium, Lavender, Lemongrass, Myrtle, Peppermint, Pine, Rose, Rosemary, Rosewood, Ylang Ylang	Bath, Massage, Vaporization, Inhalation
Headaches	Chamomile, Lavender, Lemongrass, Peppermint, Rosewood, Rosemary	Bath, Massage – apply to temples, back of neck, forehead, Diffuse or inhale directly.
Head Lice	Bergamot, Eucalyptus, Geranium, Lavender, Lemon, Tea Tree	Scalp massage, rinse
Herpes	Chamomile, Lavender, Myrrh, Tea Tree	Bath, Massage, Compress, Direct application
High Blood Pressure	Bergamot, Chamomile, Fennel, Frankincense, Lavender, Mandarin, Marjoram, Neroli, Rose, Sandalwood, Vetiver, Ylang Ylang	Bath, Massage – apply on location or on feet and hands, Diffuse or inhale directly.
Hives	Tea Tree, Peppermint, Roman Chamomile, Ravintsara, Patchouli	Apply and massage topically on location

Immune System Support	Oregano, Tea Tree, Clove, Ravintsara, Thyme, Eucalyptus, Cinnamon, Rosemary, Peppermint, Lemon, Myrtle	Apply topically to thymus, chest, back or sinuses or bottoms of feet. Warm Compress. Diffuse or inhale directly.
Indigestion	Dill, Fennel, Parsley, Peppermint, Mandarin	Massage, Inhalation.
Inflammation	Frankincense, Tea Tree, Eucalyptus, Oregano, Thyme	Apply topically on location or back or neck and massage. Diffuse or inhale water vapors.
Insect repellent	Citronella, Patchouli, Lavender, Clove	Apply to feet or exposed skin and massage or mist to skin. Also can be diffused.
Lungs (healthy function)	Eucalyptus, Frankincense, Peppermint, Lemon, Oregano	Diffuse or inhale directly, or apply topically to chest, throat and back.
Memory	Rosemary, Peppermint, Frankincense, Lemon, Clove	Diffuse or inhale directly. Or it can be applied directly to temples, crown of head or back of neck.
Muscle Cramps	Lemongrass with Peppermint, Marjoram, Rosemary	Can be applied topically on location. Massage or Bath.
Nausea	Bergamot, Black Pepper, Chamomile, Fennel, Ginger, Grapefruit, Lavender, Mandarin, Orange, Peppermint, Rosewood	Vaporization, Inhalation. Can be applied to feet, temples, stomach or wrist. Or taken in capsule.
Parasites	Oregano, Thyme, Fennel, Roman Chamomile, Lemon	Take one capsule internally. Or can be applied as warm compress to abdomen and feet.
PMS	Clary Sage, Tarragon, Fennel, Geranium, Lavender	Apply on abdomen, lower back, shoulders or feet. Massage and place a warm compress.

Seasonal Discomforts	Lavender, Lemon, Roman Chamomile, Peppermint	Can be taken in capsule, diffuser or inhaled, or applied topically on sinuses and bottoms of feet.
Shock	Peppermint, Helichrysum, Tea Tree, Roman Chamomile	Can be inhaled or diffused, or applied topically on neck, feet or over heart.
Sinusitis	Chamomile, Lavender, Eucalyptus, Lemon, Lemongrass, Myrtle, Niaouli, Peppermint, Pine, Tea Tree	Massage, Bath, Vaporization, Inhalation
Skin Irritation	Lavender, Roman Chamomile, Elemi, Tea Tree	Apply topically on location
Skin Issues	Lavender, Frankincense	Apply topically on location
Sore Throat	Basil, Black Pepper, Cinnamon, Lavender, Tea Tree, Oregano, Eucalyptus, Lemon	Can be diffused or inhaled, applied topically on throat or feet.
Sprains	Chamomile, Lavender	Massage, Bath, Compress
Stress	Lavender, Lemon, Ylang Ylang, Frankincense, Bergamot	Can be diffused or inhaled, applied topically to neck, back or bottoms of feet.
Toothache	Clove, Tea Tree, Roman Chamomile	Apply topically on location or along jawbone. Place warm compress on jawbone.
Warts	Frankincense, Tea Tree, Oregano, Clove	Apply topically on location

AROMATHERAPY MASSAGE

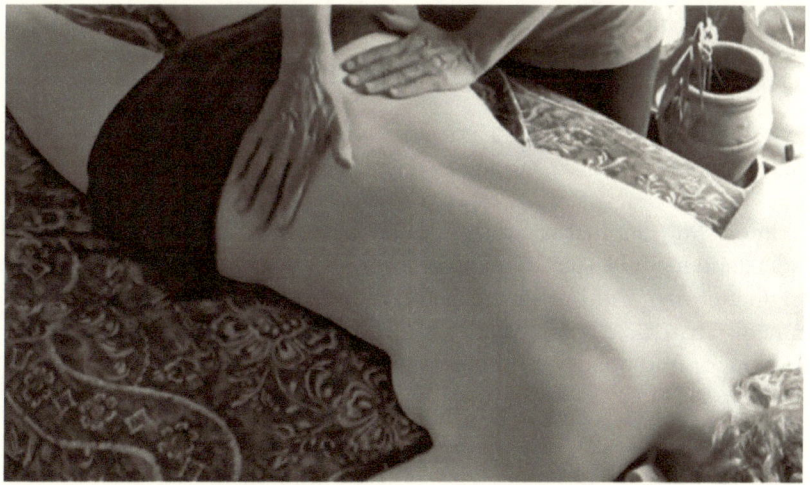

A very common way that essential oils are used is via aromatherapy and massage. There are many added benefits to using the oils this way, as shown by this **list of positives** below:

- Improves mobility by easing back pain.
- Reduces maternity stays by relaxing and soothing expectant mothers during childbirth.
- Moderates dependence on pharmaceutical medication.
- Supports the immune system by stimulating your natural network of defense: lymph flow.
- Helps rejuvenate tight, atrophied, or weak muscles.
- Boosts recovery from, and preparation for, athletic workouts.
- Enhances skin health and its overall condition.

- Improves flexibility in your joints.

- Reduces anxious or depressed feelings.

- Supports regeneration of body tissue regeneration, works to reduce your stretch marks and scar tissue.

- Improves circulation, enhances flow of oxygen and nutrients to organs and tissues.

- Alleviates swelling and adhesions from surgery.

- Relaxes cramping and spasms by easing muscles that are tired, injured, and overused.

- Boosts the body's inherent painkillers by promoting secretion of endorphins.

- Relieves pain associated with migraines.

If you consider these benefits alongside what the oils bring you, it's easy to see why more people are turning to this method.

An interesting fact that you might not know is aromatherapy as we currently understand it got its start by accident in 1920s France. A chemist, Rene Maurice Gattefosse, had burned his hand, found no other remedy nearby, and immediately soaked it in Lavender. He was surprised at how quickly it healed the wound. Additionally, he coined the term *'aromatherapy.'*

Top 15 Essential Oils For Aromatherapy

Here is a list of the **most popular essential oils for aromatherapy** use:

Bergamot

Bergamot essential oil is an extract of the *Citrus bergamia* tree, which is native to Southeast Asia. Now it can typically be found along the Ivory Coast and in Italy. It is citrus-scented and a popular aromatherapy oil that is used in colognes and perfumes.

Bergamot is applied to combat depression, stress, anxiety, and anorexia, along with a variety of infections such as eczema and psoriasis. It is also applied for stimulating the digestive system, liver, and spleen, and uplifting those feeling tired or ill-content.

Cedarwood

Cedarwood essential oil is extracted from the *Juniperus virginiana* tree, which is native to North America. It is said to have been around for centuries; history shows that the ancient Egyptians used it and it might be one of the first extracted essential oils.

Cedarwood is woody-scented and often used to achieve a lifting of the spirit, to calm feelings of anxiety and stress. It helps alleviate skin issues and respiratory problems as well. Cedarwood can also be used to ease urinary tract infections.

Chamomile

There are two varieties of Chamomile, Roman and German. Aromatherapy and essential oils are extracted from both, and the medicinal properties are different between the two. In general, Chamomile is known for having soothing characteristics (especially when applied as a tea). The essential oil is extracted from the flowering plant's leaves.

There are medicinal properties that are consistent between Roman and German chamomile, unless specifically noted. Both contain analgesic properties and offer help in eradicating acne, but the German chamomile is better at fighting inflammation in instances of digestive and urinary tract issues. Chamomile offers antidepressant, antiseptic, antibiotic, and powerful calming properties.

Eucalyptus

Eucalyptus essential oil is extracted from the eucalyptus tree, which is native to Australia. The oil has a powerful, recognizable scent and is effective against respiratory issues and diseases. It is also a diuretic, deodorant, decongestant, stimulant, an antiseptic, and an antispasmodic.

In addition, it is used to enhance concentration and applied to fight fevers, muscle pains and aches, and migraines due to its cooling properties.

Jasmine

Jasmine essential oil is an extract of *Jasminum grandiflorum*, which is an evergreen native to China. This expensive oil has powerful medicinal properties and helps ease issues associated with a range of maladies, from depression to pain during childbirth. Jasmine oil is most known for having relaxing properties.

Jasmine has been known to enhance libido, reduce stress and tension, ease respiratory problems, and relieve addiction symptoms.

Lavender

Lavender essential oil is one of the most popular oils on the market. Aptly, the plant's name has Latin roots in the word *lavera*, which translates to "to wash." It has a clean aroma and is effective at relieving stress. Lavender also works to combat the flu, colds, and migraine symptoms.

Lavender's healing effects can be attributed to the following medicinal properties: sedative, antiseptic, diuretic, antidepressant, deodorant, anti-inflammatory, and decongestant.

Lemon

Lemon essential oil is a favorite among aromatherapy enthusiasts. This oil has a fresh scent but also gets a lot of appreciation for its ability to clean almost any surface. It offers a variety of therapeutic qualities that include easing symptoms of arthritis and acne, enhancing concentration, and supporting digestion health.

Lemon oil is a natural immunity booster that helps with circulation, skin irritation, digestion problems; alleviating fever and headaches, improving mood, and reducing cellulite.

Marjoram

Marjoram essential oil has therapeutic properties to calm anxiety and hyper-activity. Add a few drops to a humidifier, vaporizer, diffuser, or warm bath. Marjoram was another popular plant among the Greeks for use in medicines; the same properties apply today. For one, it's known for helping with diges-tion issues like cramps and constipation.

Marjoram also combats stress, depression, fatigue, and circulatory and respir-atory issues.

Patchouli

Patchouli essential oil is widely known and typically associated with hippies or earthy types. It's thought that they use it because of the mood-lifting prop-erties. The oil is an extract of the plant *Pogostemon cablin* and works as an ef-fective skin-care agent.

Patchouli promotes overall skin health and cellular growth when applied top-ically. Patchouli also relieves depression, anxiety, fatigue; reduces bloating and cellulite, and curbs addiction.

Peppermint

Peppermint essential oil is often used to improve focus and alertness due to its refreshing, cooling effect. This perennial herb contains natural energy-boosting properties.

Peppermint oil offers several therapeutic properties; among them, its effect as a cooling agent can enhance mood, combat irritation and redness, assist in digestion, improve attention and focus, and alleviate congestion symptoms.

Rose

Rose essential oil is a powerful treatment within aromatherapy against issues that women, alone, often face. Roses have a long history of being distilled for essential oil extracts. Rose oil tends to be more expensive than other oils due to the quantity of roses necessary for distillation.

Rose oil is an ideal essential oil because it can help alleviate a handful of conditions and illnesses: circulation issues, depression, heart problems, anxiety, digestion issues, skin irritation, and respiratory conditions to name a few.

Rosemary

Rosemary essential oil is a powerful aromatherapy oil. There is a long history of this herb being considered sacred. It is a natural mental stimulant, can give your spirit a lift, and boost your memory.

This stimulating oil offers antidepressant, analgesic, antiseptic, antibiotic, and digestive properties. It's most known for the following health benefits: improving focus and brain performance, soothing aches and cramped muscles, easing migraines and headaches, alleviating liver and digestive infections, and promoting skin health.

Sandalwood

Sandalwood essential oil is instantly recognizable by its woody aroma. Sandalwood is an expensive oil because of the time it takes, preferred 80 years, for a tree to reach proper maturity. This is the best time to distill the essential oil, when the tree will produce maximum return and carry its strongest fragrance. This oil provides several aromatherapy benefits.

Sandalwood oil can alleviate chest pain, act as an agent of relief for tension, create a calming environment for yoga practitioners, reduce inflammation, hydrate the skin, and support mucous membranes found in the chest wall and urinary tract.

Tea Tree

Tea Tree essential oil is easily one of the most effective and popular oils for aromatherapy use. This clean-smelling oil is known to combat infection and enhance immune system function. It is known for working fast and having several uses.

This oil offers an abundance of healing properties. It combats three different kinds of infection; heals burns, skin conditions, and cuts; and repels insects. Additionally, it will soothe and treat muscle aches, cold sores, the flu, respiratory conditions, dandruff, and athlete's foot.

Ylang Ylang

Ylang Ylang essential oil is recognized by its distinct fragrance. It has a sweet aroma that is excellent for enhancing libido and reducing stress.

This extract's calming properties are the strongest, but Ylang Ylang can also soothe nausea, headaches, skin conditions; fight intestinal problems, promote hair growth, and lower high blood pressure.

Aromatherapy Facts
That You Should Know

Here are some facts about aromatherapy that are very useful to know:

1. **Essential oils are a plant's extracted essence.**

   Essential oils have therapeutic properties because they originate from a plant's vital essence. These oils are protective elements for the plant, hindering external threats like disease, pests, or even climatic changes. Current research is finding these oils can be functional in the same way for humans.

2. **Treatment with essential oils is a personalized process.**

   One scent will not work the same way for everyone. Body chemistry, if you are prone to fever, acidity, anxiety, ulcers, headaches, or anger, for instance, changes from person to person. What might be calming for you might cause sensitization or irritation in another person.

3. **Remember that less is more.**

   Essential oils are potent extracts with overpowering aromas that can overwhelm you and others. We recommend using only the amount you need or what has been directed by your therapist. Using too much oil won't speed up recovery; apply the oils you need when you need them, not just because you have them.

4. **Aromatherapy is being tested internationally to improve efficiency.**

   Business firms in Japan have tested how pumping Lemon, Jasmine, and Lavender aromatherapy oils through the air-cooling ducts would improve employee efficiency. The potential is there to reduce employee error, boost morale, and increase productivity when it is low.

5. **Aromatherapy oils could be used in public places to hinder transfer of airborne infections.**

   Because aromatherapy oils have antiseptic, antibacterial, and antiviral properties, they could be used to improve public health. Vaporizing or diffusing them in hospitals or crowded places could put these air-purifying properties to good use.

6. Further research is being conducted on aromatherapy oils.

Respected universities and hospitals all over the globe are researching the use of aromatherapy oils to validate their effectiveness and the benefits they could provide from personalized treatments.

TOP 30 ESSENTIAL OILS

This chapter is going to examine some of the very best essential oils for common ailments, in greater detail. Of course, there are thousands of essential oils – and which of these will suit you is very individual – so this list of 30 oils is just to get you started.

Always remember to speak to a health professional for advice before taking any of the essential oils.

1. Ginger

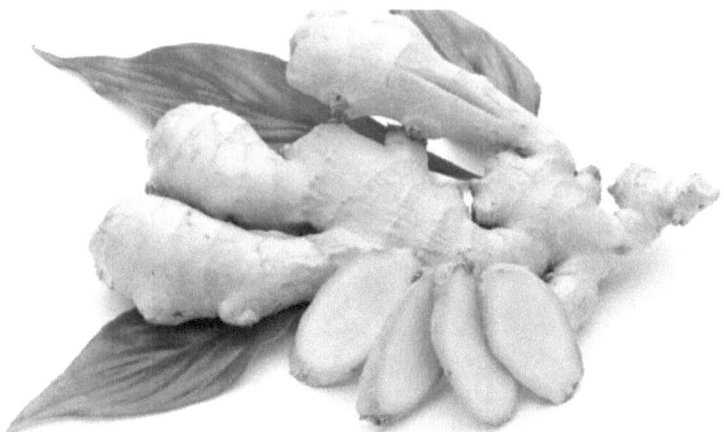

Ginger essential oil is extracted from the perennial herb's aromatic, distinctly shaped rhizome. Ginger is a member of the Zingiberaceae flowering-plant family and grows up to 4 feet high, displaying narrow leaves with a spear shape, yellow or white flowers, and small tuberous roots with brown skin that may be thick or thin. The color of the rhizome's flesh varies between yellow, white, and red.

This spicy, energizing root has been praised for centuries, boasting medicinal and culinary properties, particularly among the ancient Greek, Chinese, and Indian civilizations. Especially Ayurveda, where ginger is considered a key herb.

Latin Name: Zingiber officinale.

Color: Light yellow.

Scent: Warm, spicy, earthy, woody.

Location: Asia, West Africa.

Part of the Plant Used: Roots.

Distillation Method: The straight steam method.

Primarily Used For: Ginger is brilliant for pregnancy – it's often recommended for morning sickness due to its ability to settle stomach problems and nausea. It's also very effective in case of premenstrual syndrome.

TIP: When applied topically, it may help relieve Arthritic Knee Pain and Rheumatoid Arthritis symptoms.

Other Uses: Colic, Constipation, Diarrhea, Indigestion, Motion Sickness, Nausea, Respiratory issues, Arthritis.

Application Method: Aromatically, topically or internally.

Where To Buy: Local specialist or online resources, such as Amazon.com, iHerb.com, YoungLiving.com, MountainRoseHerbs.com.

Notes: Avoid topical use with children under 2. Do not take if using warfarin, diabetes medication, heart medication or aspirin. May cause sensitivity to the skin.

2. Lavender

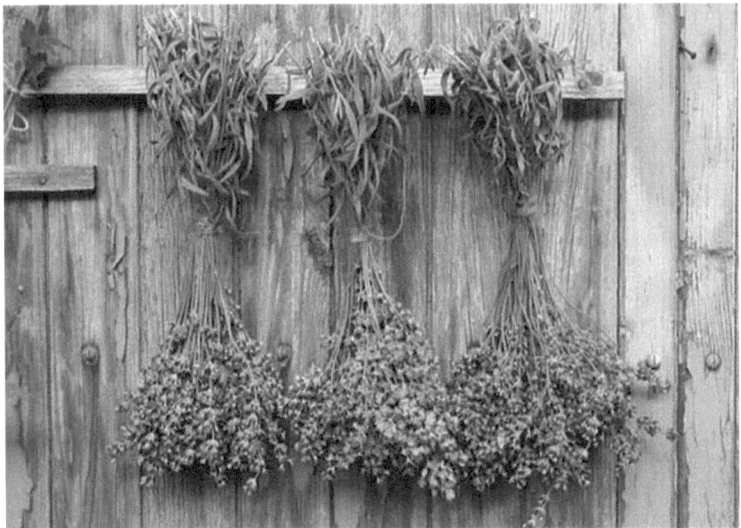

Lavender is an evergreen plant within the mint family. This fragrant perennial is a native of southern Europe, and Bulgaria, France, Tasmania, and Spain grow most of the world's commercial crop. A flourishing industry is getting its start in Norfolk, England. Individual plants can grow as tall as 3 ft, showing leaves that appear narrow, downy, and grey. The blue-grey flowers bloom from tall, slender stems.

Lavender's oil can be released from its star-shaped hairs by rubbing a flower or leaf right between your fingers. Making its health benefits, such as antiseptic and anti-inflammatory properties, practically tangible. Those same properties make Lavender essential oil perfect for treating bug bites, minor burns, and even anxiety, depression, insomnia, and restlessness.

Latin Name: Lavandula angustifolia.

Color: Clear with a tinge of yellow.

Scent: Floral, fresh, sweet, herbaceous and sometimes fruity.

Location: Primarily Tasmania.

Part of the Plant Used: Flowers, buds and leaves.

Distillation Method: The straight steam method.

Primarily Used For: Lavender is well known for its stress reliving properties. It's extremely calming and mood enhancing.

TIP: For headaches or allergic reactions, apply 1 drop of oil to sinuses or forehead. For restlessness or insomnia, rub the bottom of your feet with a couple drops. For skin irritation, rub diluted Lavender oil on the area of concern 3 times per day.

Other Uses: Sleep Aid, Insect Bites/Stings, Burns, Bruises, Cuts, Scrapes, Hay Fever, Growing Pains, Acne, Dry Skin, High Blood Pressure, Pet Smells, Soap Replacement, Allergies.

Application Method: Aromatically or topically.

Where To Buy: Local specialist or online resources, such as Amazon.com, YoungLiving.com, doTerra.com.

Notes: Suitable for children, but only in very loses doses.

3. Peppermint

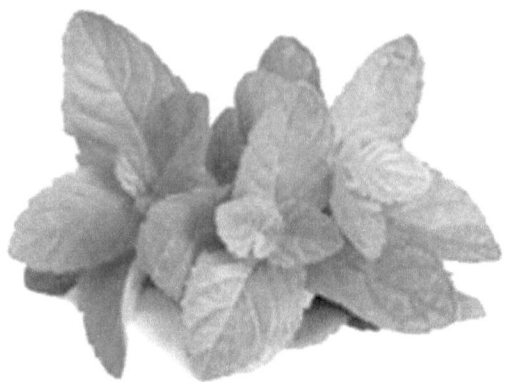

Peppermint is a perennial herb and a hybrid of spearmint and watermint. The plant is indigenous to Europe and the Middle East, but can typically be grown wherever it is placed – favoring moist locales. It does not produce seeds but spreads via growth of its rhizomes. The regions that once cultivated peppermint for its oil, such as New Zealand, the Great Lakes region of the United States, and the Galapagos Islands, now consider it invasive because feral plants now grow in abundance.

The health benefits of Peppermint essential oil include improving digestion and relieving pain associated with irritable bowel syndrome, enhancing skin health, easing headaches, and alleviating cold and flu symptoms.

Latin Name: Mentha piperita.

Color: Clear with a yellow tinge.

Scent: Strong, minty.

Location: Europe, Asia.

Part of the Plant Used: Ariel parts.

Distillation Method: The straight steam method.

Primarily Used For: Peppermint is brilliant for treating all sorts of digestive disorders.

TIP: Peppermint is also very efficient for treating headaches. Apply 1-2 drops of essential oil diluted with carrier oil and massage it onto your forehead and the back of your neck or temples.

Other Uses: Fever, Headache, Joint Pain, Memory Recall, Sinus Congestion, Stomach Discomforts, Cooling Sore Feet, Energy, Allergies, Ticks, Spiders.

Application Method: Aromatically, topically, or internally

Where to Buy: Local specialist or online resources, such as Amazon.com, YoungLiving.com, iHerb.com, MountainRoseHerbs.com.

Notes: Do not take if you're suffering from gallbladder disease or achlorhydria. Avoid during pregnancy or breastfeeding. Avoid use with children under 6.

4. Cinnamon

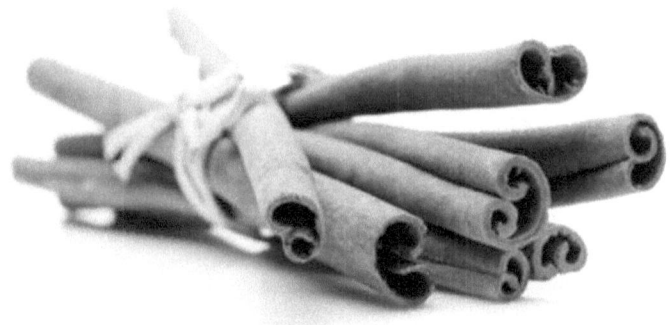

Cinnamon, a name that applies to nearly a dozen tree species, is also the name of a spice product extracted from the inner bark of trees from the genus Cinnamomum. All of the trees are members of the Cinnamomum genus within the Lauraceae family. Only a few, though, are grown for commercial spice purposes. Most cinnamon available is derived from a species, "cassia," that is only related to the species known as "true cinnamon." Popular in cooking, the spice is used for both savory and sweet dishes.

The health benefits of Cinnamon include decreasing the risk of heart disease, enhancing your body's sensitivity to insulin, and lowering blood sugar; this is supported by these properties: being anti-inflammatory, an antioxidant, and antimicrobial.

Latin Name: Cinnamomum zeylanicum.

Color: Golden yellow to brown.

Scent: Richer aroma than ground cinnamon.

Location: Asia.

Part of the Plant Used: Leaf or bark.

Distillation Method: The straight steam method.

Primarily Used For: Cinnamon oil is regularly used for lifting mood and enhancing life but can also be a perfect remedy to fight influenza.

TIP: Ease the pain of a sore throat by adding 1 drop of Cinnamon oil to hot water or tea.

Other Uses: Sore Throat, Cold, Indigestion, Increases Brain Activity, High Blood Pressure, Mosquitoes, Removes Blood Impurities, Viral Infections, Ulcers.

Application Method: Aromatically, topically, internally.

Where to Buy: Local specialist or online resources, such as Amazon.com, iHerb.com, YoungLiving.com, doTerra.com.

Notes: Suitable for children, but only in very low doses. Do not take if using blood-thinners such as Warfarin. Also avoid it if you experience prostate problems.

5. Frankincense

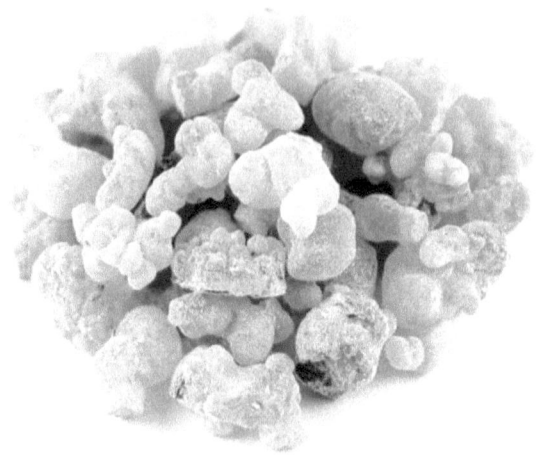

Frankincense essential oil is extracted from Boswellia genus trees, specifically *Boswellia carteri* and *Boswellia sacra*. Boswellia trees are known to grow in Arabian and African regions, including Ethiopia, Yemen, Somalia, and Oman. In fact, Oman is the most ancient, and best known, source of frankincense. Regions like India, China, and the Mediterranean have been importing it from there for centuries. The Boswellia tree's milky sap is extracted directly from the bark, which is given several days to harden into a gum resin. Then, the resin is scraped off in tiny, firm droplets.

This extract's health benefits include reducing stress and negative feelings, boosting immunity, and enhancing overall skin health; those benefits are promoted by these medicinal properties: astringent, disinfectant, antiseptic, digestive, and diuretic. Frankincense has long been considered a valuable herbal supplement; in Biblical times, it was considered **more valuable than gold**!

Latin Name: Boswellia.

Color: Light yellow.

Scent: Fresh, woody, balsamic, mildly spicy, fruity.

Location: Africa, Arabia.

Part of the Plant Used: Resin.

Distillation Method: The straight steam method.

Primarily Used For: When it comes to beauty and skin care, frankincense has always been recommended due to its antifungal properties. It can also help to build and maintain a healthy immune system.

TIP: It can help to fade scars from acne, stretch marks, and surgery. You can also apply 1 drop of Frankincense oil to wounds to clean and disinfect. Try also using Frankincense oil to get rid of warts, moles, or skin tags.

Other Uses: Inflammation, Infections, Pain Relief, Asthma, Anxiety, Depression, Seizures, Cancer, Skin Issues, Warts, Parkinson's Disease, Tumors, Alzheimer's Disease, Bites (Insects, Snakes), Antiaging.

Application Method: Topically to the affected area, internally, or aromatically.

Where to Buy: Local specialist or online resources, such as Amazon.com, iHerb.com, YoungLiving.com, NativeAmericanNutritionals.com.

Notes: Suitable for children, but only in very low doses.

6. Sandalwood

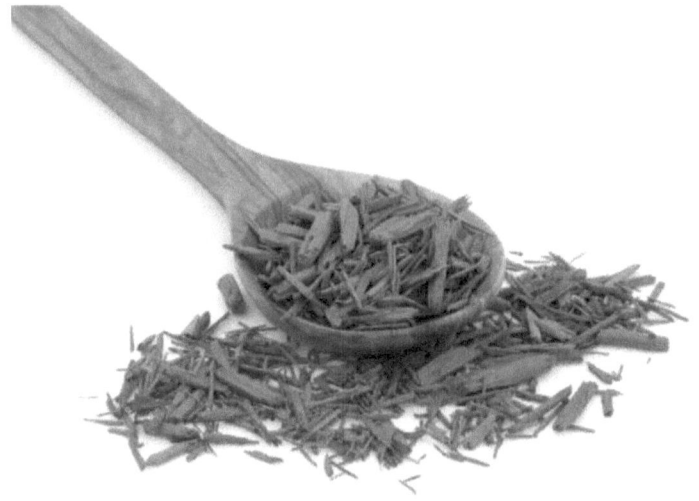

Sandalwood essential oil is extracted from the wood of mature sandalwood trees via steam distillation. "Mature" trees are between 40 and 80 years old. It's suggested to wait until the tree's 80th year for extraction because more oil will be available, and it will give off a stronger aroma.

The health benefits of this aromatic extract include enhancing mental clarity, acting as a natural aphrodisiac, and producing a relaxed and calm emotional state; those benefits can be attributed to these medicinal properties: expectorant, antiseptic, hypotensive, anti-inflammatory, memory enhancer, antispasmodic, sedative, astringent, emollient, cicatrisant, disinfectant, carminative, tonic, and diuretic.

Latin Name: Santalum album.

Color: Clear to pale yellow.

Scent: Rich, sweet, fragrant, woody, floral.

Location: Europe, India, Asia.

Part of the Plant Used: Wood.

Distillation Method: The straight steam method.

Primarily Used For: This essential oil is famous for helping to recreate youthful skin, as it tones and relieves itching, inflammation, and dehydrated skin.

TIP: Apply up to 2 drops of Sandalwood directly to your face, drape a towel over your head, and hold it over a bowl of steaming water to replicate a spa-style steam facial. Your skin will feel nourished and rejuvenated.

Other Uses: Acne, Candida, Immune Stimulant, Cold Sores, Back Pain, Calming, Scar Tissue, Skin Issues, Stress, Respiratory Infections, Insomnia, Cancer, Insect Repellent.

Application Method: Topically to the affected area, internally, or aromatically.

Where to Buy: Local specialist or online resources, such as Amazon.com, iHerb.com, YoungLiving.com, MountainRoseHerbs.com.

Notes: Suitable for children, but only in very low doses.

7. Elemi

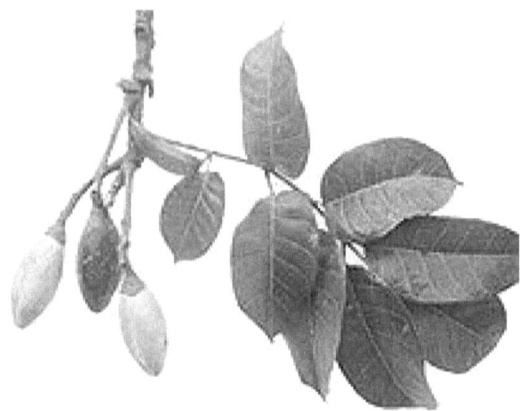

Elemi is a tree native to the Philippines, from which the oleoresin that is extracted is also known as elemi. This pale-yellow substance has a consistency similar to honey. Elemi essential oil is distilled from the resin via the steam method. It is fragrant with a scent that combines elements of lemon and sharp pine.

The health benefits of Elemi essential oil are alleviating extreme coughing, bronchitis, stress, wrinkled skin, wounds, scars, and catarrh. Similar to those of frankincense, elemi contains the medicinal properties of being antiseptic, expectorant, analgesic, tonic, and stimulant. In fact, elemi is the same botanical family as frankincense and is also known as *"Poor Man's Frankincense."*

Latin Name: Canarium luzonicum.

Color: Clear with a tinge of yellow.

Scent: Fresh, citrusy, peppery, spicy.

Location: Philippines.

Part of the Plant Used: Resin.

Distillation Method: The straight steam method.

Primarily Used For: Elemi is known for its energy-boosting, anti-fatigue properties, and also greatly improves skin condition.

TIP: Use elemi to virtually erase facial scars, even those that you've had a long time. In just a few days, the scarred skin will appear more even compared to the rest of your face. After one week, smaller scars can completely disappear, while deeper scars will become harder to see.

Other Uses: Skin Issues, Rashes, Muscle Pain, Bronchitis, Stress, and Anxiety.

Application Method: Aromatically and topically.

Where to Buy: Local specialist or online resources, such as Amazon.com, YoungLiving.com, EdensGarden.com, HopeWellOils.com.

Notes: Suitable for children, but only in very low doses.

8. Roman Chamomile

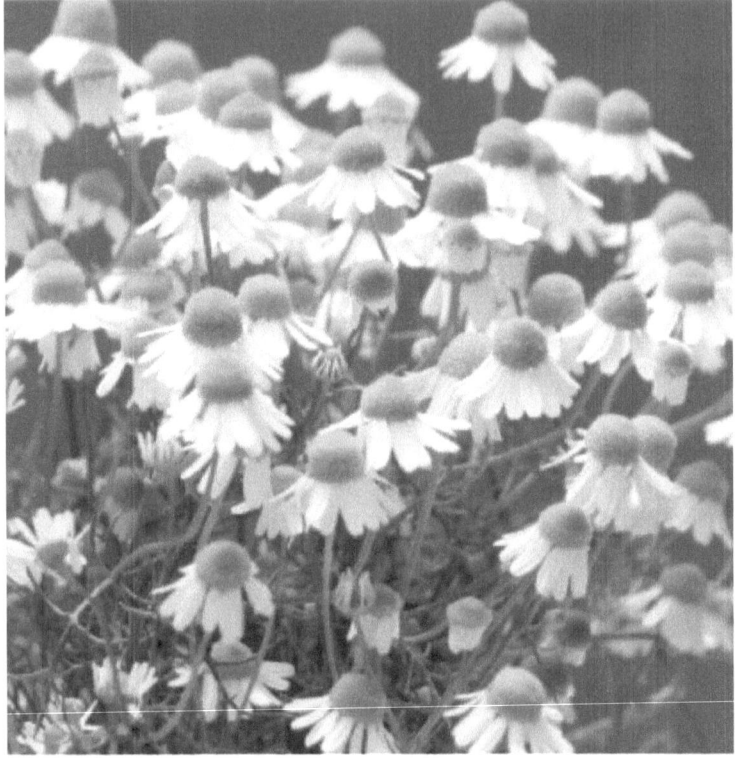

Roman chamomile blooms with daisy-like white flowers and has a sweet, fruity, herbaceous fragrance. Some of its medicinal properties are being anti-inflammatory, an antispasmodic, digestive, antiseptic, and antibiotic. The essential oil's health benefits include alleviating premenstrual syndrome symptoms, promoting skin health, easing insomnia, and reducing feelings of depression and anxiety.

Latin Name: Chamaemelum nobile.

Color: Grey or very pale blue.

Scent: Bright, crisp, sweet, fruity, herbaceous.

Location: Northwestern Europe, North Ireland.

Part of the Plant Used: Flowers.

Distillation Method: The steam distilled method.

Primarily Used For: Roman chamomile contains chemicals that can cause sedation which makes it perfect for anyone struggling to sleep.

TIP: Roman chamomile helps to detoxify the blood and liver. Use 1 drop in 8 oz of water or apply 3 drops on the liver area.

Other Uses: Insomnia, Anxiety, Depression, Skin Conditions, ADHD, Shock, PMS Relief, Digestive Problems, Acne, Allergies, Teeth Pain, High Blood Pressure.

Application Method: Aromatically, topically, or internally.

Where to Buy: Local specialist or online resources, s such as Amazon.com, YoungLiving.com, NativeAmericanNutritionals.com, HopeWellOils.com.

Notes: Suitable for children, but only in very low doses. Do not take if you're using sedatives, blood thinners, pain killers or allergic to ragweed. Avoid if pregnant or nursing.

9. Grapefruit

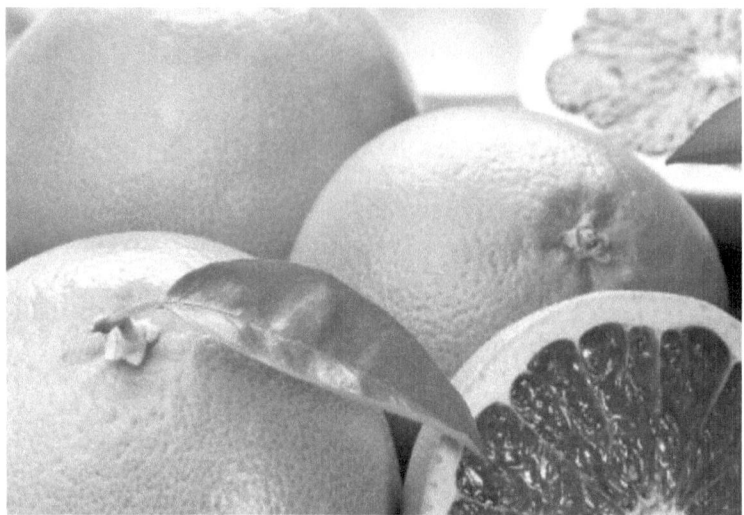

Grapefruit and its essential oil are excellent sources of Vitamin C. Foods rich in Vitamin C can boost immunity and alleviate cold symptoms. Vitamin C also provides anti-inflammatory properties and so can reduce symptoms associated with inflammatory conditions, such as osteoarthritis, rheumatoid arthritis, and asthma. Grapefruit is known to have antidepressant and stimulating properties that can make you feel better and more alert. This essential oil can keep hunger in check, helping you lose weight or maintain your current weight; reduce stress, hinder the progression of gum disease, and promote heart health. Due to its being a great source of Vitamin C, this essential oil is known to decrease the risk of kidney stones, stroke, and cancer.

Latin Name: Citrus paradisi.

Color: Pale yellow to yellow.

Scent: Citrusy, sweeter more concentrated smell of grapefruit.

Location: Barbados.

Part of the Plant Used: Peel.

Distillation Method: Cold pressed.

Primarily Used For: Grapefruit oil is highly spoken about by new moms because it's brilliant for reducing stretch marks and tightening skin.

TIP: Want to lose weight? Put 2-4 drops in a glass of water before meals to help calm appetite.

Other Uses: Weight Loss, Cravings, Addiction, Cleansing, Depression, Hair Tonic, Kidney Cleansing, Anorexia, Cellulite, Antiaging.

Application Method: Topically to the affected area, internally, or aromatically.

Where to Buy: Local specialist or online resources, such as Amazon.com, iHerb.com, YoungLiving.com, doTerra.com.

Notes: Suitable for children, but only in very low doses. When applied topically, it is important to avoid sunlight for a minimum of 6 hours.

10. Lemon

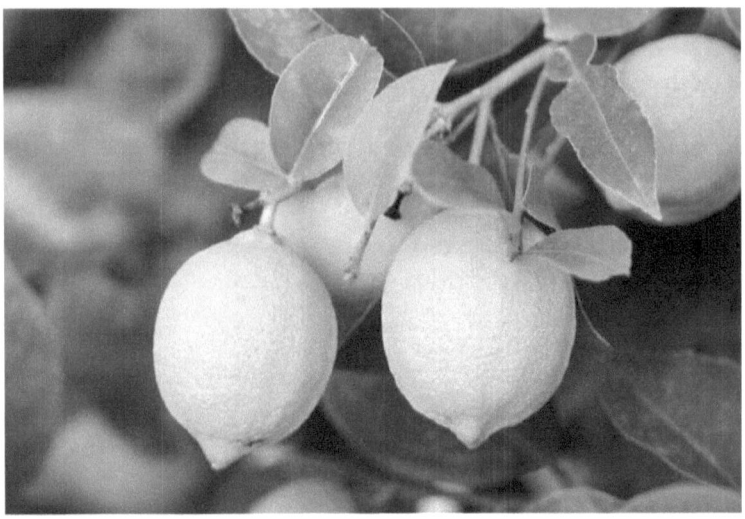

Lemons grow on a small evergreen tree native to Asia. This distinctive yellow fruit has been used across the globe for cooking and non-cooking purposes. Primarily the lemon is used for its juice, but the rind and pulp are also popular and commonly used ingredients. Lemon juice contains about 6% citric acid, which is responsible for the sour taste. Lemon essential oil's most notable health benefits include promoting weight loss, supporting healthy immune system function, regulating sleep and relieving stress, and treating stomach disorders.

Latin Name: Citrus limon.

Color: Pale to dark yellow.

Scent: Fresh concentrated lemon.

Location: Asia.

Part of the Plant Used: Peel.

Distillation Method: Cold pressed.

Primarily Used For: Lemon oil is brilliant for hair care. It works well no matter what your hair type.

TIP: Use Lemon essential oil around the house to help remove stains from laundry; sticky messes like gum, glue, or adhesives; oil and grease spots, and crayon from almost every surface.

Other Uses: Energy, Allergies, Anxiety, Asthma, Bad Odors, Warts, Sore Throat, Disinfectant, Gout, Digestive Aid, Skin Care, Hangover, Detox Liver.

Application Method: Topically to the affected area or Aromatically.

Where to Buy: Local specialist or online resources, such as Amazon.com, YoungLiving.com, iHerb.com, HopeWellOils.com.

Notes: Avoid topical use for children under 2. When applied topically, it is important to avoid sunlight for a minimum of 6 hours.

11. Spearmint

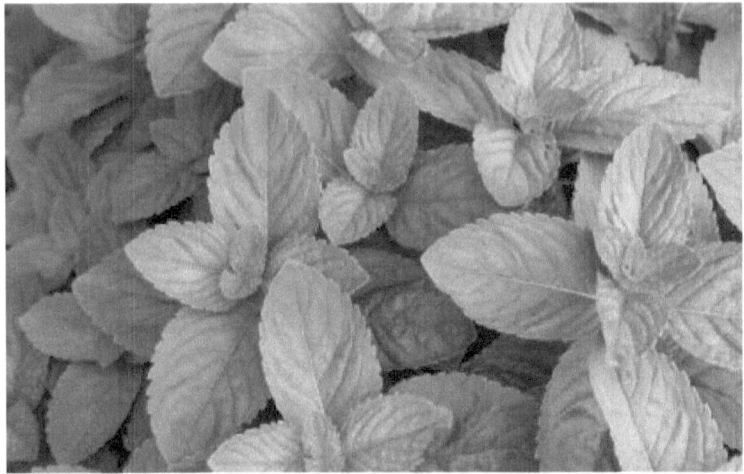

Spearmint is a perennial herb originating from the Mediterranean. Its use dates back to ancient times, extensively in Greece. From Ayurvedic medicine, it was known to enhance digestion, ease headaches, and alleviate skin problems. It could brighten teeth, fight sexually transmitted diseases, medicate mouth sores, and was frequently added to baths. Today, Spearmint essential oil is still applied to alleviate digestive discomfort, nausea, and painful symptoms of menstruation.

Latin Name: Mentha spicata.

Color: Clear.

Scent: Minty and slightly fruity.

Location: Europe, Asia.

Part of the Plant Used: Leaves, flowers, and buds.

Distillation Method: The straight steam distilled method.

Primarily Used For: Spearmint essential oil has carminative, antiseptic, restorative, and antispasmodic medicinal properties. It is very often used to help with headaches.

TIP: Add 1-2 drops to any dessert, drink, salad for flavoring and to promote digestion.

Other Uses: Asthma, Disinfectant, Improves Concentration, Mosquito Repellent, Stress, Wounds and Ulcers, Menstrual Pain, Bronchitis, Digestive Disorders, Eczema, Bad Breath.

Application Method: Aromatically, topically, or internally.

Where To Buy: Local specialist or online resources, such as Amazon.com, iHerb.com, YoungLiving.com, NowFoods.com.

Notes: Suitable for children, but only in very low doses. Avoid during pregnancy or breast feeding.

12. Eucalyptus

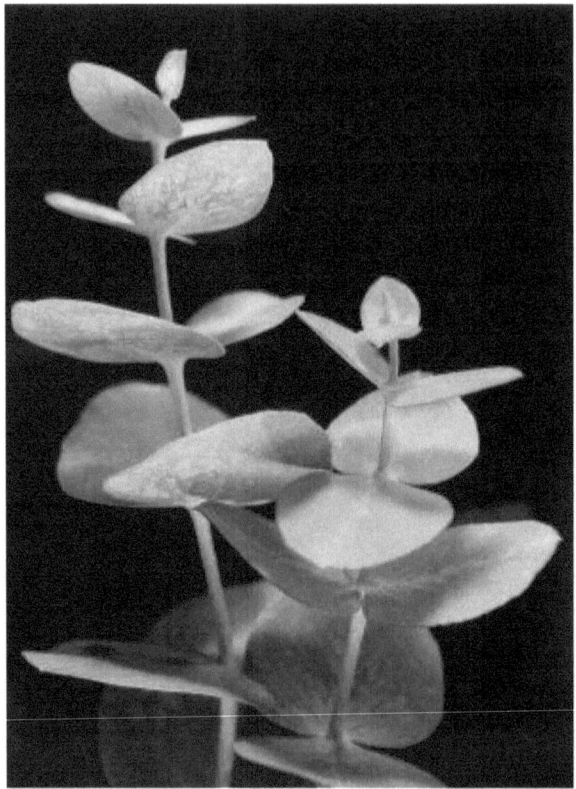

Eucalyptus essential oil acts like almost any other volatile oil. Even though it's colorless and has a recognizable odor and taste, it has not been popular for use in aromatherapy. Little was known about it until recently, unlike its ancient aromatherapy counterparts.

However, Eucalyptus oil's health benefits are far-reaching. Its medicinal properties include being anti-inflammatory, antiseptic, stimulating, antibacterial, an antispasmodic, a deodorant, and a decongestant. Far-reaching health benefits, including relieving muscle pain, improving hair health, and fighting flu symptoms, have attracted the world's attention and provoked a great deal of research into how its usage will offer benefits for the worlds of aromatherapy and conventional medicine.

Latin Name: Eucalyptus Radiata.

Color: Clear.

Scent: Fresh, medicinal, earthy, woody.

Location: Australia, Indonesia, Philippines.

Part of the Plant Used: Leaves.

Distillation Method: The straight steam method.

Primarily Used For: Eucalyptus is famous for its soothing properties which make it the perfect oil for foot care. It is also highly effective for respiratory infections.

TIP: Use drops of Eucalyptus oil to freshen the air with a diffuser or add to the bottom of the tub before taking a shower.

Other Uses: Respiratory Congestion, Asthma, Hay Fever, Bronchitis, Sinus Infection, Herpes Simplex, Lice, Sore Muscles, Arthritis, Skin Disorders, Insect Repellent, Stress, Wounds, Cuts, Burns or Ulcers, Intestinal Parasites.

Application Method: Topically to the affected area or aromatically.

Where to Buy: Local specialist or online resources, such as Amazon.com, YoungLiving.com, EdensGarden.com, iHerb.com.

Notes: Avoid use with children under 10. Avoid higher doses, and always dilute with carrier oil for topical application.

13. Myrrh

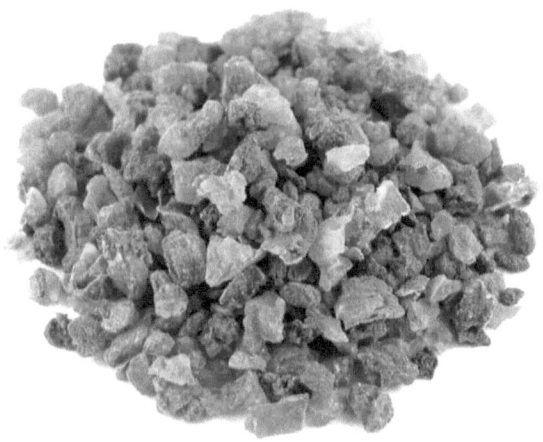

Myrrh gum, similar to frankincense, is the aromatic oleoresin extracted from various small, thorny tree species within the genus Commiphora. Myrrh resin is harvested by "wounding" the trees to "bleed" them of this yellowish, waxy gum. It quickly coagulates, then hardens and becomes glossy – with age, white streaks appear as it darkens beyond the clear, opacity it has upon harvesting.

This well-known gum resin has a long history of being applied as a medicine, perfume, and incense. It has also been ingested by mixing with wine. Myrrh's health benefits include boosting immunity, helping skin remain youthful, enhancing circulation, and alleviating pain; these benefits are attributed to its medicinal properties: antifungal, astringent, antiseptic, stimulant, antispasmodic, antimicrobial, and anti-inflammatory.

Myrrh was mentioned in the Bible 17 times!

Latin Name: Commiphora molmol.

Color: Golden yellow or brown.

Scent: Warm, earthy, woody, balsamic.

Location: Yemen.

Part of the Plant Used: Resin.

Distillation Method: The straight steam method.

Primarily Used For: Being antiseptic and anti-inflammatory, Myrrh is often applied for its abilities to enhance oral health and relieve body pain.

TIP: Improve oral health and get your teeth cleaner by adding up to 2 drops of Myrrh oil to your current toothpaste.

Other Uses: Respiratory Congestion, Menstrual Disorders, Cancer, Diabetes, Immune Support, Chapped Skin, Wrinkles, Ulcers, Fungal Infections, Allergies, Gum Infections, Hyperthyroidism, Inflammation.

Application Method: Topically, aromatically, or internally.

Where to Buy: Local specialist or online resources, such as Amazon.com, YoungLiving.com, MountainRoseHerbs.com, EdensGarden.com.

Notes: Suitable for children, but only in very low doses. Avoid during pregnancy or breast feeding. Always dilute this thick oil before application.

14. Rosemary

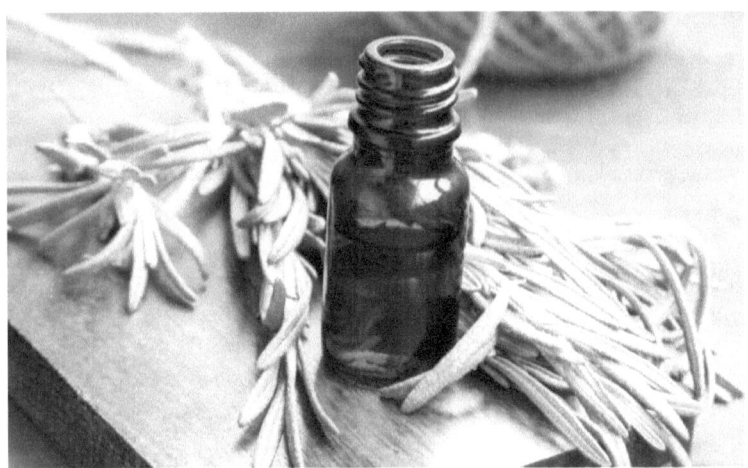

Rosemary's name has roots in the Latin words *ros* ("dew") and *marinus* ("sea"), or "dew of the sea." There is also a story that claims the Virgin Mary spread a blue cloak over a shrub as she rested; afterward, the white flowers turned blue. The plant was then known as the "Rose of Mary." The herb looks like lavender and is related to mint, displaying leaves that resemble flat pine needles highlighted with silver. Its woodsy, citrusy aroma has become a staple in many gardens, kitchens, and apothecaries.

The Egyptians, Greeks, Romans, and Hebrews considered Rosemary sacred, and in the Middle Ages, people used it to protect against the bubonic plague and ward off evil spirits.

Latin Name: Rosmarinus officinalis.

Color: Clear.

Scent: Fresh, herbaceous, sweet, slightly medicinal.

Location: Mediterranean.

Part of the Plant Used: Leaves, flowers, and buds.

Distillation Method: The straight steam method.

Primarily Used For: The scent of Rosemary oil is sharp and camphorous and has been shown to enhance proscriptive memory, which is the ability to remember things happening in the future. There have been some scientific studies that found that diffusing Rosemary while studying can increase long-term memory by 75%.

TIP: Rub Rosemary essential oil on bottoms of feet or stomach to help with digestion.

Other Uses: Alzheimer's Disease, Asthma, Bronchitis, Hepatitis, Herpes, Liver Disorders, Mental Clarity, Pain Relief, Digestive Problems, Headaches, Baldness, Throat and Sinus Infections, Cold and Flu, Gallbladder Complaints, Fibromyalgia.

Application Method: Aromatically, topically or internally.

Where to Buy: Local specialist or online resources, such as Amazon.com, iHerb.com, YoungLiving.com, NowFoods.com.

Notes: Avoid use with children under 6. Do not take if you have an allergy to aspirin; suffer from bleeding disorders, epilepsy, high blood pressure, ulcers, colitis or if you're pregnant, breastfeeding, or trying to conceive.

15. Clove

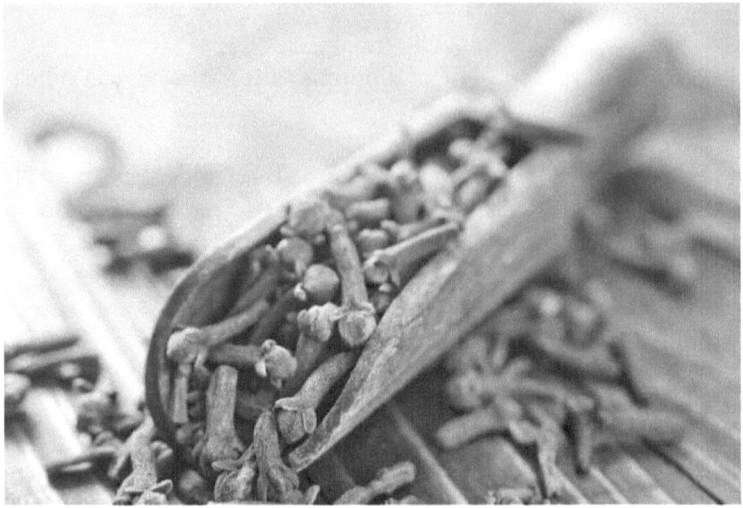

Clove trees are native to the Indonesian Maluku Islands. These evergreen trees are part of the family Myrtaceae, display big leaves and clustered red flowers, and grow to nearly 12 m tall. Cloves are the aromatic flower buds from this tree, which are generally used as a spice. Cloves are primarily grown and harvested in Tanzania, Indonesia, Sri Lanka, India, Zanzibar, and Madagascar.

Clove essential oil is most known for being a very powerful antioxidant. Some of its other medicinal properties include improving skin health, indigestion; relieving asthma and cough, headache, toothache, and stress.

Latin Name: Syzygium aromaticum.

Color: Golden yellow to brown.

Scent: Spicy, warm but slightly bitter, woody, richer than clove buds.

Location: Indonesia.

Part of the Plant Used: Buds.

Distillation Method: The straight steam method.

Primarily Used For: Clove oil is anti-inflammatory and antimicrobial and is often used to relieve the symptoms of the common cold.

TIP: Add 1 drop to toothpaste to promote oral health, or apply 1 drop to soothe teeth or gums.

Other Uses: Nausea, Toothache, Teething, Hypothyroidism, Cuts, Wounds, Skin Cancer, Oral Infections, Premature Ejaculation, Stress, Diabetes, Insect and Bug Repellent, Digestion Issues, Herpes, Warts, Fungal Infections.

Application Method: Aromatically, topically or internally. Avoid use of high doses, and always dilute with carrier oil for topical application.

Where to Buy: Local specialist or online resources, such as Amazon.com, YoungLiving.com, doTerra.com, iHerb.com, TheHealthBay.com.

Notes: Avoid use with children under 2. Do not use if allergic to eugenol, suffering from Crohn's disease, or have liver problems. Avoid use of cloves and Clove oil during pregnancy.

16. Oregano

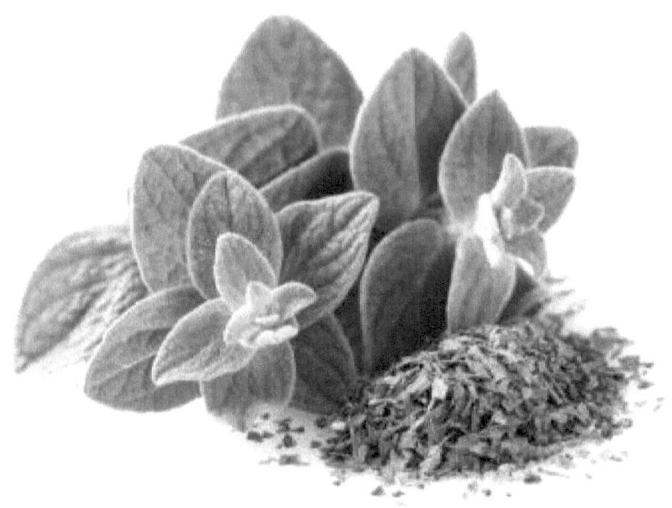

Oregano is a hardy, perennial herb and another member of the mint family. The essential oil is extracted from the herb's flowers and leaves. The plant is native to Europe, however, now it can be grown in a variety of regions across the globe. This bushy plant displays dark, green leaves up to 3 cm in length and can get as tall as 35 in.

Oregano essential oil is known for being a very strong antimicrobial, and the ancient Romans and Greeks used it for a variety of medicinal purposes. It was considered a symbol of happiness, used in traditional crowns for both bride and groom during ancient wedding ceremonies. Along with fighting broad spectrum microorganisms, this oil's health benefits include being a natural antibiotic, improving digestive health, hindering allergic reaction, and promoting hair and skin health.

Latin Name: Origanum vulgare.

Color: Pale yellow.

Scent: Herbaceous, sharp.

Location: Greece, India.

Part of the Plant Used: Leaves, flowers, and buds.

Distillation Method: The straight steam method.

Primarily Used For: Oregano oil is brilliant for aiding the digestive system, ridding the body of common stomach issues.

TIP: Did you know you can use Oregano oil to get rid of your skin tags? Dab Oregano oil to dry clean skin tag several times a day. Apply for up to 2 weeks until skin tag disappears or falls off.

Other Uses: Athlete's Foot, Candida, Cold, Flu, Food Poisoning, Pain Relief, Wrinkles, Asthma, Acne, Respiratory Disorders, Immune Support, Warts.

Application Method: Aromatically, topically, or internally. Dilute with preferred carrier oil before applying directly to skin.

Where to Buy: Local specialist or online resources, such as Amazon.com, iHerb.com, YoungLiving.com, MountainRoseHerbs.com.

Notes: Avoid topical use with children under 5. Do not take if you suffer from bleeding disorders or diabetes. Avoid use in pregnancy and breast feeding.

17. Fennel

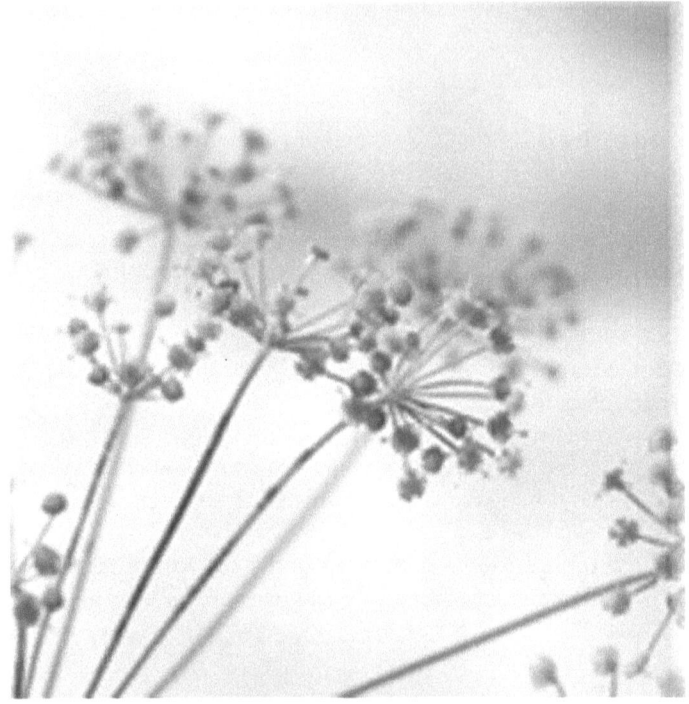

Fennel provided the ancient Romans and Egyptians several medicinal benefits. For example, this little seed boosted emotional and spiritual well-being, regulated the female reproductive system, treated bites from snakes, and supported lung and kidney function. Warriors used fennel because, spiritually, they believed they would gain longevity, strength, and courage for battle. As far back as the Medieval Age, it was believed that fennel could block a witch's spell and ward off evil spirits in general.

Today, every day, we reap similar benefits from Fennel essential oil. It assists with the occasional digestive upset and supports the glandular, respiratory, and circulatory systems.

Latin Name: Foeniculum vulgare.

Color: Clear with a faint yellow tinge.

Scent: Sweet, spicy, like licorice.

Location: Mediterranean.

Part of the Plant Used: Seeds.

Distillation Method: The straight steam method.

Primarily Used For: Fennel is known for its breath-freshening properties, so it's often used to fight halitosis.

TIP: When suffering from constipation, apply a few drops on the belly neat or diluted. Or add 1 drop to a glass of water and drink. To reduce menstrual cramps, add it to a carrier oil and massage over the lower abdomen.

Other Uses: Digestive Disorders, Constipation, Urinary Tract Disorders, Menstrual Cramps, Bruises, Cuts, Wrinkles, Cough, Intestinal Parasites, Mental Stimulant, Asthma, Rheumatism, Breast and Liver Cancer, Anemia.

Application Method: Topically, aromatically, or internally.

Where to Buy: Local specialist or online resources, such as Amazon.com, YoungLiving.com, MountainRoseHerbs.com.

Notes: Avoid use with children under 5. Avoid if suffering from epilepsy.

18. Geranium

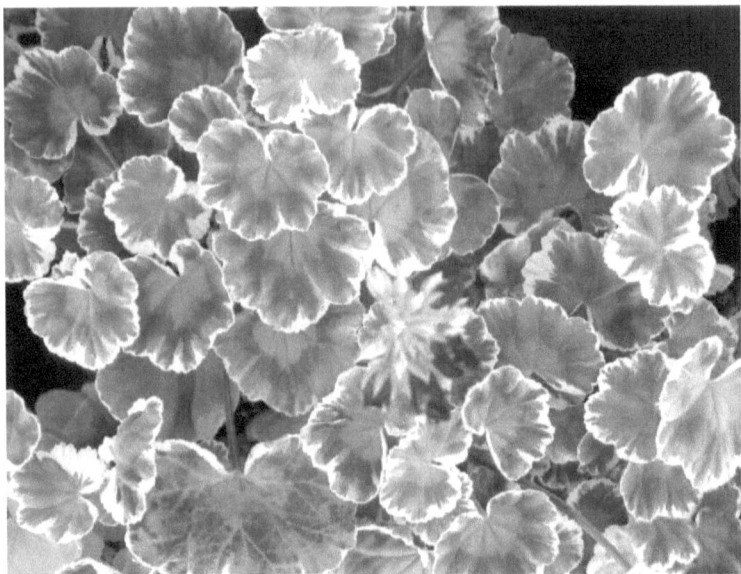

Geranium essential oil has medicinal benefits that are supported by its properties as a vermifuge, diuretic, tonic, hemostatic, styptic, cicatrisant, deodorant, cytophylactic, vulnerary agent, and an astringent. These properties are the reason this extract is a popular essential oil in aromatherapy; it offers these health benefits: reducing blood pressure, relieving depression and stress, balancing hormones, improving skin health, reducing irritation and inflammation, improving circulation, enhancing kidney function, relieving symptoms of menopause, and boosting dental health.

Latin Name: Pelargonium.

Color: Ranges from clear to amber.

Scent: Floral, fresh, sweet, slightly fruity.

Location: Eastern Mediterranean.

Part of the Plant Used: Leaves.

Distillation Method: The straight steam method.

Primarily Used For: Geranium oil functions to reduce anxiety and depression. It is a natural sedative and has the ability to lift mood.

TIP: Geranium is irreplaceable oil for women. It's a natural hormone balancer, antidepressant, aphrodisiac, skin reviver, and anti-cellulite. Minimize effects of cellulite by mixing the oil with your carrier oil of choice, then massaging it onto the area of concern. Additionally, make a bath with up to 10 drops of oil to relieve stress with tension, a headache, and premenstrual syndrome.

Other Uses: Hormone Support, Impetigo, Jaundice, Endometriosis, Dermatitis, Herpes, PMS, Thyroid Imbalance, Ringworm, Shingles, Cellulite, Headache, Respiratory Issues, Mosquito Repellent.

Application Method: Aromatically, topically, or internally.

Where to Buy: Local specialist or online resources, such as Amazon.com, iHerb.com, YoungLiving.com, HopeWellOils.com.

Notes: Suitable for children, but only in very low doses.

19. Cypress

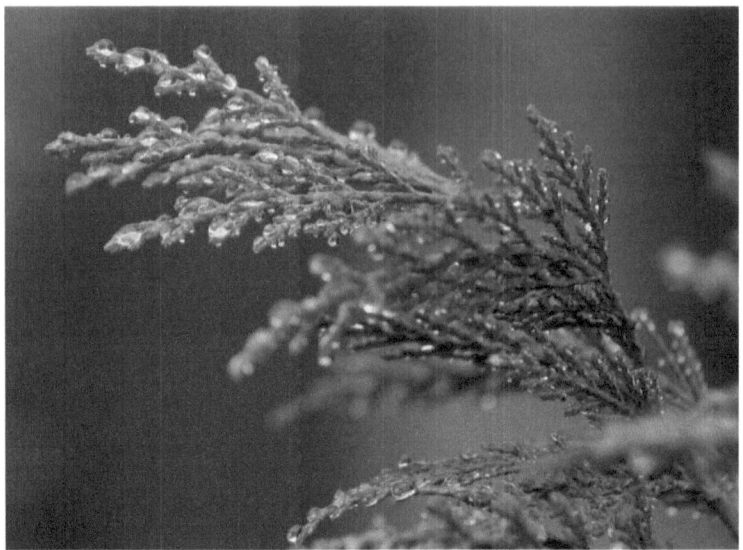

Cypress essential oil is distilled from the stems, needles, and young twigs of cypress trees via the steam method. The cypress is a needle-bearing tree native to Deciduous and Coniferous regions. The oil extracts have medicinal properties attributed to components such as Linalool, Alpha Pinene, Terpinolene, Beta Pinene, Myrcene, Alpha Terpinene, Sabinene, Bornyl Acetate, Cadinene, Carene, Cedrol, and Camphene. Despite its close association with death, mainly for being seen in so many cemeteries, this extract is known for its ability to alleviate some devastating illnesses.

The well-known health benefits of this extract are supported by these properties: diuretic, astringent, deodorant, antiseptic, hemostatic, antispasmodic, vasoconstricting, hepatic, sedative, styptic, respiratory tonic, and sudorific.

Latin Name: Cupressaceae.

Color: Pale yellow.

Scent: Fresh, herbaceous, woody.

Location: Southeast USA.

Part of the Plant Used: Needles.

Distillation Method: The straight steam method.

Primarily Used For: Cypress oil is an antispasmodic. It's perfect for preventing spasms.

TIP: Diffuse, inhale, or gargle at the first sign of throat discomfort. Add 1-2 drops to toner to help reduce oily skin conditions.

Other Uses: Asthma, Hemorrhoids, Menstrual Problems, Sore Throat, Varicose Veins, Edema, Lymphatic Decongestant, Internal and External Wounds, Diabetes, Arthritis, Stroke, Cold and Cough, Respiratory Congestion, Anxiety, Stress, Muscle Cramps, Kidney or Liver Problems.

Application Method: Aromatically or topically.

Where to Buy: Local specialist or online resources, such as Amazon.com, YoungLiving.com, doTerra.com, iHerb.com, NowFoods.com.

Notes: Do not use on very young children. Avoid during pregnancy or breastfeeding.

20. Lemongrass

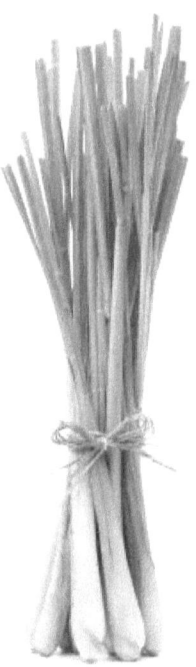

Lemongrass is a plant with therapeutic, antimicrobial, antibacterial, rubefacient, and antioxidant properties, which classifies it as a broad-spectrum remedy. Because it is generally used in Asian cooking, it is often available in the grocery store, at a health food store, from an online store, or in an ethnic store. Lemongrass produces medicinal benefits whether you use the essential oil or steeped leaves for tea.

The aromatic compound, citral, which is often called lemonal, is Lemongrass's main component. Citral is antimicrobial, antifungal, and helps the body use Vitamin A. This is the compound that gives lemongrass its lemon scent, and accounts for it being used so frequently in perfumes. Besides being aromatic, it contains pheromonal properties, making it perfect for insect repellant. Additional compounds Nerol, Geraniol, and Myrcene boost its fragrance, Geranyl Acetate boosts its natural flavor, and Citronella is a known insecticide.

Latin Name: Cymbopogon.

Color: Pale to vivid yellow.

Scent: Fresh, lemony, earthy.

Location: Asia.

Part of the Plant Used: Grass.

Distillation Method: The straight steam method.

Primarily Used For: Lemongrass oil is a tonic in a very clear sense. Its anti-pyretic properties make it great for fighting off fevers.

TIP: Add Lemongrass oil to drinking water for kidney disorders and infections. Can also be taken in capsules or added to water daily to reduce high cholesterol.

Other Uses: Cancer, Stress, Muscle and Joint Pain, Bladder Infection, Insect Repellent, Ligaments, Salmonella, Varicose Veins, High Cholesterol, Kidney Disorders, Digestion Disorders, Athlete's Foot, Acne.

Application Method: Aromatically, topically, or internally.

Where to Buy: Local specialist or online resources, such as Amazon.com, iHerb.com, YoungLiving.com, MountainRoseHerbs.com.

Notes: Avoid topical use for children under 2. May irritate sensitive skin. Avoid during pregnancy or breastfeeding.

21. Cajeput

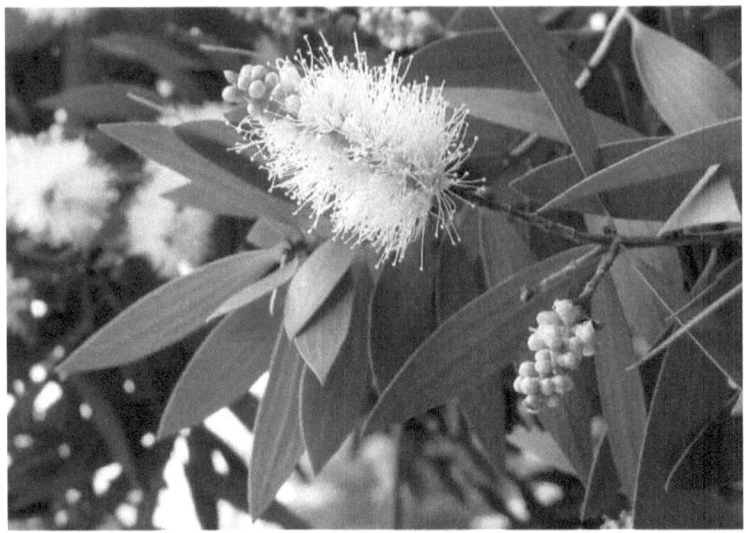

Cajeput essential oil is obtained from the myrtaceous trees Melaleuca cajuputi, Melaleuca leucadendra, and likely others found throughout Maritime Southeast Asia and across warmer parts of the Australian continent. However, most of the oil is actually made on Sulawesi, an Indonesian island – where the tree gets its name "kayu putih" meaning "white wood." The extract is distilled from leaves collected during a hot day, macerated with water, and allowed to ferment overnight.

This oil has a pungent odor similar to mixing camphor and turpentine. It's a volatile oil that can be applied internally for uses similar to Clove oil, applied externally for use as a counterirritant, and appears in sore muscle liniments and traditional Indonesian medicine.

Latin Name: Melaleuca leucadendron.

Color: Clear with a yellow tinge.

Scent: Fresh, camphorous aroma with a fruity note.

Location: Indonesia.

Part of the Plant Used: Leaves.

Distillation Method: The straight steam method.

Primarily Used For: Due to the chemical cineole, Cajeput oil is primarily used for pain relief. Cineole may cause irritation or warmth when applied directly to the skin.

TIP: You can use Cajeput essential oil to tackle infestations of parasites. Especially fleas, brush your cat or dog weekly and add 1-2 drops of the oil to your pet's brush bristles.

Other Uses: Fever, Insect Repellent, Neuralgia, Muscle and Joint Pain, Intestinal Worms, Chest Infections.

Application Method: Topically to the affected area or aromatically.

Where to Buy: Local specialist or online resources, such as Amazon.com, EdensGarden.com, MountainRoseHerbs.com, doTerra.com.

Notes: Avoid use with children under 6. Avoid during pregnancy or breast-feeding. Can irritate sensitive skin.

22. Ravensara

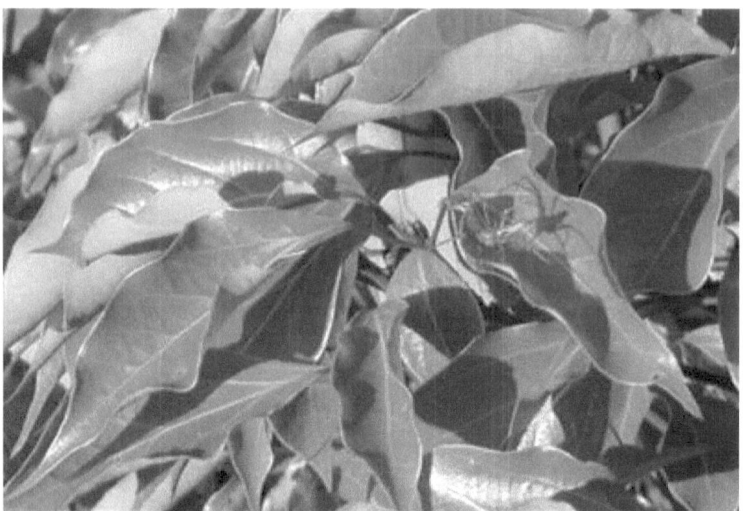

Ravensara essential oil is extracted from the large rainforest tree native to the mysterious island of Madagascar, just off Africa's eastern coast. This powerful extract is praised as being a cure-for-all on the same level as Australia's Tea Tree essential oil.

This extract's health benefits are supported by these properties: aphrodisiac, analgesic, antiviral, antiallergenic, antispasmodic, antibacterial, antiseptic, antimicrobial, antifungal, antidepressant, disinfectant, tonic, diuretic, relaxant, and expectorant.

Latin Name: Ravensara aromatica.

Color: Clear with a tinge of yellow.

Scent: Slightly medicinal, sweet with a fruity hint.

Location: Madagascar.

Part of the Plant Used: Leaves.

Distillation Method: The straight steam method.

Primarily Used For: Ravensara oil has analgesic properties, which makes it great for pain relief and joint care. It's often used for earache.

TIP: Ravensara oil facilitates absorption of nutrients in the body and helps treat improper blood and lymph circulation.

Other Uses: Respiratory Issues, Sexual Dysfunction, Toothache, Headache, Warts, Herpes, Athlete's Foot, Shingles, Immune Support.

Application Method: Topically to the affected area or aromatically.

Where to Buy: Local specialist or online resources, such as Amazon.com, doTerra.com, MountainRoseHerbs.com.

Notes: Suitable for children, but only in very low doses. Avoid during pregnancy or breastfeeding.

23. Immortelle (Helichrysum)

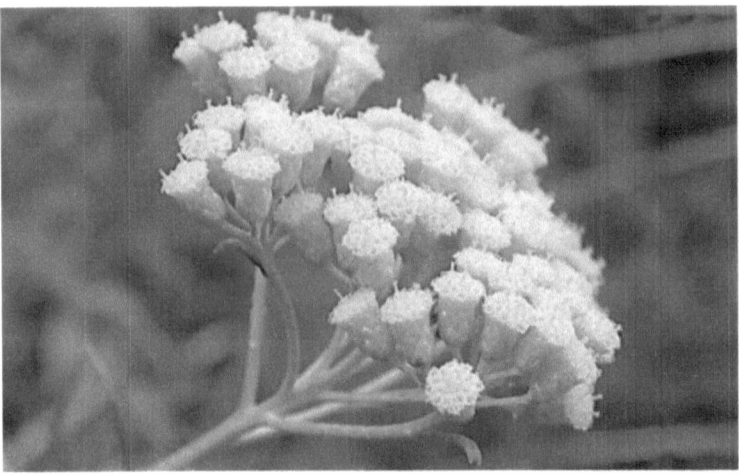

Helichrysum essential oil is distilled from the plant's flowers and produced mostly in the Mediterranean countries of France and Madagascar. The earthy, rich, warm oil has analgesic, regenerative, and anti-inflammatory properties, which makes it perfect for healing formulas that treat muscle pain, liver problems, arthritis, respiratory infection and inflammation and working as a detoxifier in substance withdrawal.

Latin Name: Xerochrysum bracteatum.

Color: Light yellow.

Scent: Fresh, earthy, herbaceous.

Location: Mediterranean.

Part of the Plant Used: Flowers.

Distillation Method: The straight steam method.

Primarily Used For: Immortelle is useful skin-care oil, it being antiallergenic, anti-inflammatory, and astringent. It promotes new cell growth and has good antioxidant qualities making it a brilliant anti-wrinkle cream. Simply add 1 drop to face cream before applying.

TIP: Due to its tissue-regeneration properties, it's recommended to apply helichrysum to cuts, burns, scrapes, wounds, scars, and bruises.

Other Uses: Earache, Blood Clots, Hearing Loss, Scars, Varicose Veins, Nose Bleeding, Tinnitus, Stretch Marks, Cuts, Bruises, Burns, Thyroid Issues, Eczema, Psoriasis, Cough, Digestion Issues, Pain Relief, Stress.

Application Method: Topically to the affected area, aromatically or internally.

Where to Buy: Local specialist or online resources, such as NativeAmericanNutritions.com, MountainRoseHerbs.com, EdensGarden.com.

Notes: Do not use with children under 2 years old. Always dilute if pregnant or breastfeeding. To be avoided after surgery.

24. Tea Tree (Melaleuca)

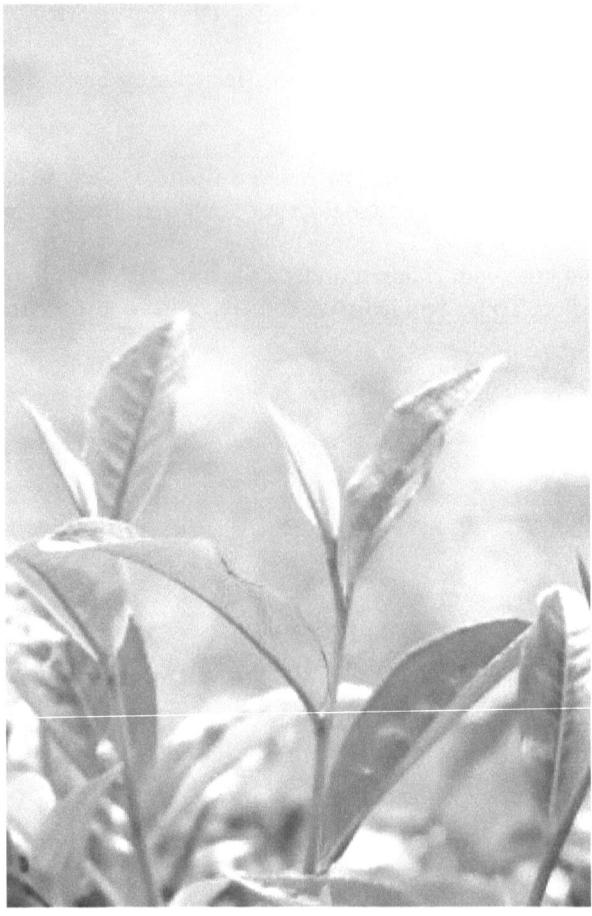

Tea Tree essential oil is considered one of the most popular healing extracts. This oil is extracted from the *Melaleuca alternifolia* plant, or the tea plant, via steam distillation of the leaves and twigs – this is not the plant that produces tea leaves used in the popular beverage. This particular tea tree hails from Australia, New South Wales and South East Queensland specifically. Because its impressive qualities are so well-known now, it can easily be found in other parts of the world.

This extract's health benefits are supported by these properties: antiviral, antibacterial, antiseptic, antimicrobial, expectorant, balsamic, fungicide, cicatrisant, sudorific, insecticide, and stimulant.

Latin Name: Melaleuca alternifolia.

Color: Clear with a yellow tinge.

Scent: Medicinal, earthy, woody, herbaceous, fresh.

Location: Australia.

Part of the Plant Used: Leaves.

Distillation Method: The straight steam method.

Primarily Used For: The cicatrisant property of this essential oil makes it heal wounds quickly and protects them from infections. Furthermore, it can help neutralize or diminish the scar marks and after spots left by eruptions, boils, pox, and acne.

TIP: Use a few drops of Tea Tree oil in a DIY household cleaner for added germ killing. It can also be applied after piercings to avoid infection.

Other Uses: Athlete's Foot, Canker/Cold Sores, Herpes, Cavities, Gum Diseases, Allergies, Earache, Lice, Warts, Eczema, Candida, Wounds, Respiratory Issues, Sore Throat, Ringworm, All-purpose Cleaner, Laundry Refresher, Mold, Mites, Toothache, Ticks, Dandruff.

Application Method: Topically to the affected area or aromatically.

Where to Buy: Local specialist or online resources, such as Amazon.com, iHerb.com, YoungLiving.com, EdensGarden.com.

Notes: Avoid topical use with children under 2. May irritate sensitive skin. Always dilute if pregnant or breastfeeding.

25. Coriander

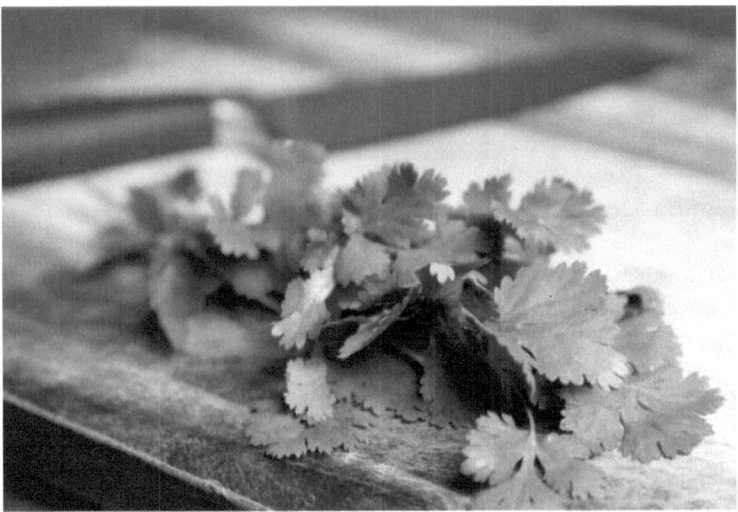

Coriander essential oil is extracted by steam distillation from the plant's seeds. This essential oil has medicinal properties attributed to compounds such as Phellandrene, Borneol, Pinene, Terpinolene, Cineole, Linalool, Cymene, Terpineol, and Dipentene.

The health benefits of the Coriander extract are supported by these properties: antispasmodic, analgesic, carminative, aphrodisiac, deodorant, depurative, fungicidal, digestive, stimulant, lipolytic, stomachic, and stimulant.

Latin Name: Coriandrum sativum.

Color: Pale yellow.

Scent: Sweet, herbaceous, woody, spicy, slightly fruity.

Location: Southern Europe, Northern Africa, Southwestern Asia.

Part of the Plant Used: Seeds.

Distillation Method: The straight steam method.

Primarily Used For: Coriander promotes the breaking down, or hydrolysis, of cholesterol and fat, which is also known as lipolysis. When the process of lipolysis speeds up, that means you lose weight faster.

TIP: Boost digestion by rubbing a few drops on your stomach after eating or applying the oil internally.

Other Uses: Stress, Depression, Detoxification, Fungal Infections, Digestive Disorders, Toothache, Muscle and Joint Pain, Libido, Bad Mouth Odor, Migraines, Measles, Diarrhea, Arthritis, Diabetes, Eczema, Ulcers.

Application Method: Aromatically, topically, or internally. Can cause sensitivity to the skin when used topically.

Where to Buy: Local specialist or online resources, such as Amazon.com, iHerb.com, YoungLiving.com, MountainRoseHerbs.com.

Notes: Avoid use with very young children. Do not take if you suffer from low blood pressure or if you are allergic to mugwort, aniseed, caraway, fennel, or dill.

26. Clary Sage

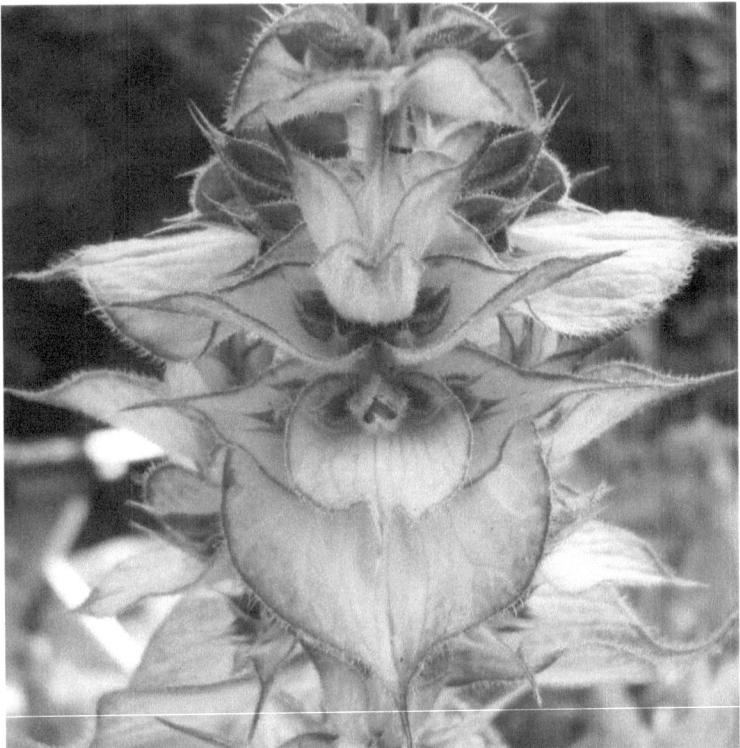

Clary Sage essential oil is extracted from the leaves and buds of the *Salvia sclarea* plant by steam distillation. This highly praised herb has long been considered medicinal, owing to its various health benefits. It is believed to be a species native to Europe; even though it's a genetic relative to common garden sage, its organic compounds are slightly different. If "Clary Sage" doesn't sound familiar, you may recognize *"Muscatel oil."* This is the common name given to Clary Sage essential oil because it has traditionally been used to make muscatel wine.

The health benefits of muscatel oil, including improving and maintaining good vision, are associated with its properties as an aphrodisiac, antidepressant, astringent, anticonvulsive, bactericidal, antispasmodic, carminative antiseptic, deodorant, nervine, digestive, sedative, emenagogue, stomachic, euphoric, uterine, and hypotensive substance.

Latin Name: Salvia sclarea.

Color: Light to golden yellow.

Scent: Earthy, warm, and herbaceous.

Location: Northern Mediterranean, North Africa, Central Asia.

Part of the Plant Used: Leaves and flowers.

Distillation Method: The straight steam method.

Primarily Used For: Clary Sage essential oil contains natural phytoestrogens. It has a mellow, warm herbal scent that is relaxing and uplifting, making it a perfect choice during PMS and for menopausal women. Use 3-5 drops in a carrier oil as a massage oil to relieve menstrual cramps.

TIP: Inhale it in deep breaths to reduce blood pressure and promote calm.

Other Uses: High Blood Pressure, Depression, Insomnia, Stress, Anxiety, Menstrual Problems, Drug Addiction, Low Libido, Muscle Pain, Dementia, Prostate Problems, High Cholesterol, Cysts, Dysentery, Skin Diseases, Anti-aging, Wounds, Ulcers, Sores.

Application Method: Topically to the affected area, aromatically, or internally.

Where to Buy: Local specialist or online resources, such as Amazon.com, YoungLiving.com, doTerra.com, iHerb.com.

Notes: Suitable for children, but only in very low doses. Avoid if pregnant or breastfeeding.

27. Cedarwood

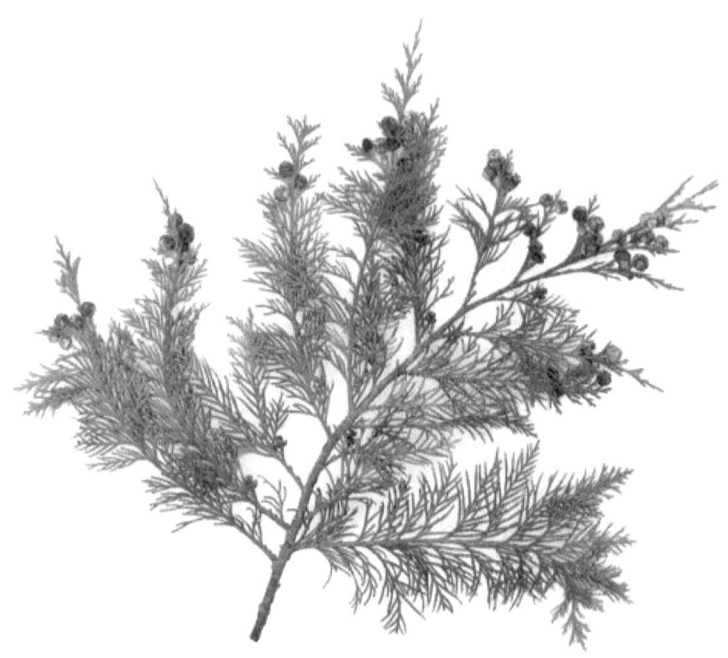

Cedarwood essential oil is derived from the roots, wood, and foliage of co-nifers in the cypress or pine botanical families. People have found uses for it within the manufacturing, medicine, perfumery, and art worlds.

There are a variety of "cedar" oils drawn from the cypress and pine families. The prominent oils from this group are distilled from juniper and cypress wood more than "true" cedars. Similarly, Cedar Leaf oil, and others like it, are extracted, pressed, or distilled from the Eastern arborvitae tree's leaves, roots, and wood.

Latin Name: Cedrus atlantica.

Color: Light to golden yellow.

Scent: Woody, sweet.

Location: North America.

Part of the Plant Used: Wood.

Distillation Method: The straight steam method.

Primarily Used For: This wonderful essential oil has many, many healing properties, but it is most often used for its tranquilizing effect. Cedarwood oil is also a valuable tool in skin issues such as dermatitis and eczema. It's best used topically, on the affected area.

TIP: To help relieve symptoms of bronchitis, rub 1-2 drops of Cedarwood essential oil on the chest. Add 1 drop to your forehead to promote good sleep.

Other Uses: Acne, Eczema, Oily Skin, Insomnia, Respiratory Issues, Anger, Anxiety, Bronchitis, Hair Loss, Mold, UTI, Mosquito and Insect Repellent, High Blood Pressure, Wounds.

Application Method: Topically to the affected area or aromatically. May cause sensitivity when applied to the skin.

Where to Buy: Local specialist or online resources, such as Amazon.com, YoungLiving.com, doTerra.com, iHerb.com.

Notes: Suitable for children, but only in very low doses.

28. Arborvitae

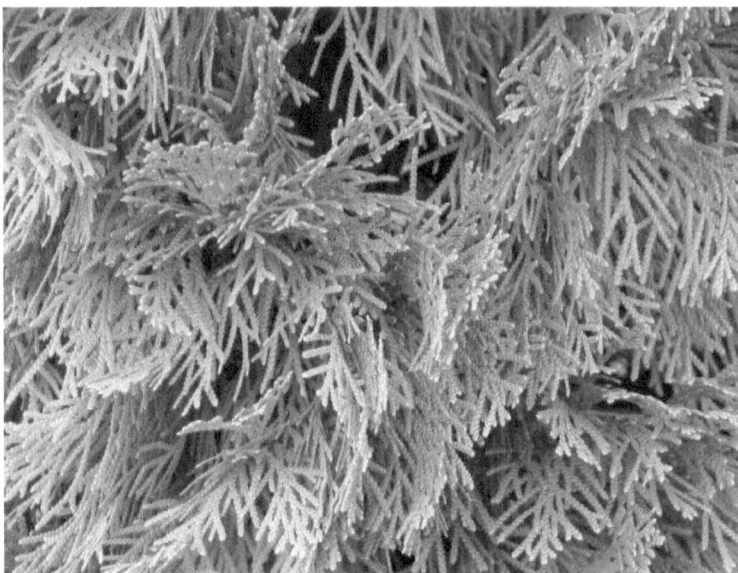

Arborvitae, as abundant in size as it is in medicinal benefits, is also called "*tree of life*." So much so, that one of these trees could be centuries old, or already dead, and still not show signs of any deterioration. This particular tree is native to Canada, and because of its inherent preservation properties, every part of the tree was used by Native Americans not only for building important day-to-day items like clothing, boats, and baskets, but also for its health benefits.

A group of chemical compounds, which Arborvitae essential oil has in abundance, called tropolones, are what protect the tree of life from seasonal and environmental threats. The tropolones support healthy cell function and provide purifying properties. One of those compounds, Thujic acid, has been researched because it is so adept at protecting against environmental threats. Another tropolone, Hinokitiol, can repel insects and maintain cell health while keeping harmful elements from affecting the body.

Latin Name: Thuja.

Color: Clear to pale yellow/green.

Scent: Pungent, woody, warm.

Location: Canada.

Part of the Plant Used: Needles and twigs.

Distillation Method: The straight steam method.

Primarily Used For: Arborvitae oil is well known for its balancing effects. It's often recommended for emotional assistance.

TIP: Did you know that Arborvitae oil was shown in studies to be 5 times more effective than Tea Tree oil against candida? Apply oil topically a couple times daily by massaging the reflex points or area of concern.

Other Uses: Eczema, Dermatitis, Fungal Infections, Insect Repellent, Cancer, Candida, Menstrual Problems, Immune System Support, Chest Congestion, and Cough.

Application Method: Aromatically, topically, or internally.

Where to Buy: Local specialist or online resources, such as Amazon.com, EdensGarden.com.

Notes: Suitable for children, but only in very low doses. Consult a doctor if pregnant or breastfeeding.

29. Thyme

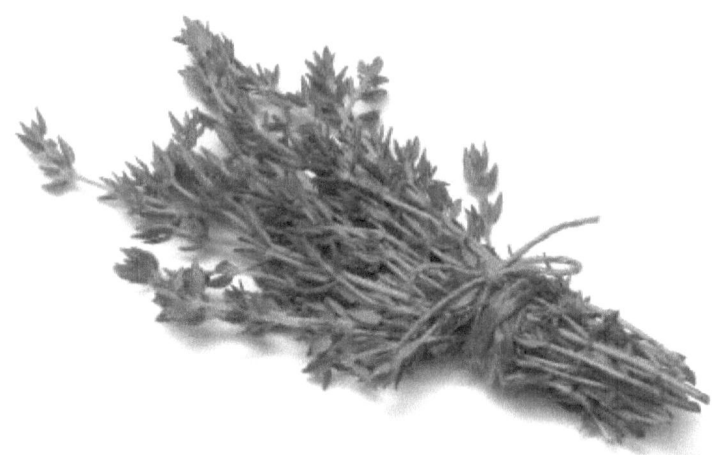

Thyme is a perennial herb used mostly in aromatherapy, potpourri, and cooking. Being related to mint, Thyme is also known for its medicinal properties, which makes it perfect for uses in ointments, elixirs, and mouthwash.

Spain, France, and Morocco are among the primary producers of Thyme essential oil, and Mediterranean countries have recognized the benefits of this oil for centuries. Additionally, it has a long history within the practice of Ayurveda.

The real takeaway about Thyme, though, is that it's known as one of the **strongest natural antiseptics**. This oil can destroy pathogenic organisms that cause bad breath, tooth decay, and gingivitis; 16 strains of fungi, and more than 60 bacteria strains.

Latin Name: Thymus vulgaris.

Color: Reddish brown.

Scent: Fresh, medicinal, herbaceous.

Location: Europe, Morocco.

Part of the Plant Used: Leaves, flowers, and buds.

Distillation Method: The straight steam method.

Primarily Used For: Thyme essential oil is perfect for toning up the circulatory system and boosting immunity.

TIP: Do you want to stop snoring? Rub 2 drops of Thyme under the feet before sleep.

Other Uses: Alzheimer's Disease, Cardiovascular Issues, Mold, Infectious Diseases, Cough/Cold, Laryngitis, Fatigue, Antiaging, Hair Loss, Psoriasis, Eczema, Intestinal Worms, Arthritis, Gout, Wounds, Digestions Disorders, Depression, Gingivitis.

Application Method: Aromatically, topically or internally. Always dilute with carrier oil for topical application.

Where to Buy: Local specialist or online resources, such as Amazon.com, iHerb.com, YoungLiving.com, EdensGarden.com.

Notes: Suitable for children, but only in very low doses. Avoid during pregnancy or breastfeeding.

30. Melissa

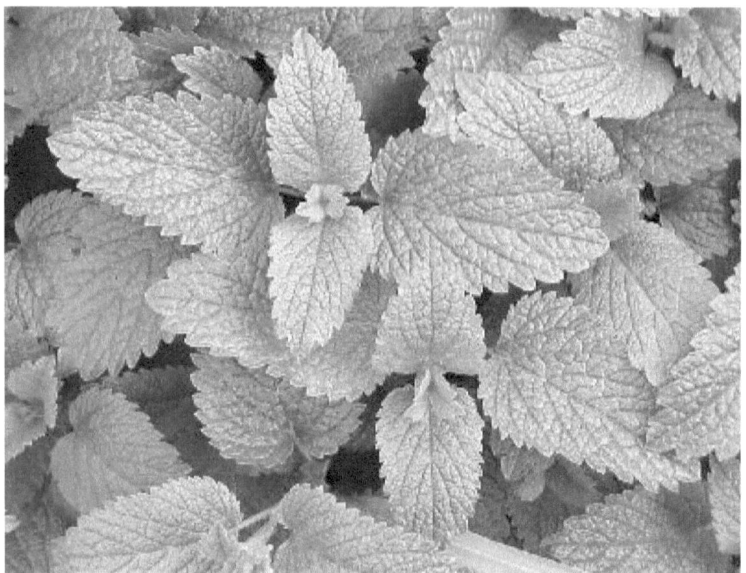

Melissa, also known as lemon balm or sweet balm, is a revitalizing plant with properties that boost the function of your immune system. It has been reported that Lemon Balm oil complements your current skin-care regimen, has antibacterial properties, and helps ease anxiety and insomnia.

Latin Name: Melissa officinalis.

Color: Yellow.

Scent: Fresh, lemony, herbaceous.

Location: South Central Europe.

Part of the Plant Used: Leaves, flowers, and buds.

Distillation Method: The straight steam method.

Primarily Used For: Melissa is best known for its work against the herpes simplex virus, including cold sores.

TIP: Diffuse at night or rub on forehead, shoulders, or chest to reduce stress and promote emotional well-being.

Other Uses: Respiration Issues, Depression, Digestive Disorders, Anxiety, Cold Sores, Insomnia, Asthma, Insect Bites, Migraines, High Blood Pressure, Fungal Infections, Immune Support.

Application Method: Internally, topically to the affected area, or aromatically. May irritate sensitive skin.

Where to Buy: Local specialist or online resources, such as Amazon.com, YoungLiving.com, EdensGarden.com.

Notes: Do not allow children under the age of 12 to take. Always consult a doctor before using it. Avoid if pregnant or breastfeeding.

Please remember while reading this, **that everyone is individual, and your treatment should be treated as such.** Just as a variety of traditional medication can be tried to see what suits you, you will need to experiment with essential oils.

It is advisable to speak to other essential oil users, and online forums are a great way to do that. Here are a couple of examples to get you started:

My Essential Oils Forum at *myessentialoilsforum.com*

Auroma Forum at *auroma.forumchitchat.com*

For safety, don't take the oils internally – at the very least, not until you are very experienced – and *always* seek medical advice from a health professional before trying any of the recommended oils.

ESSENTIAL OILS TO AVOID

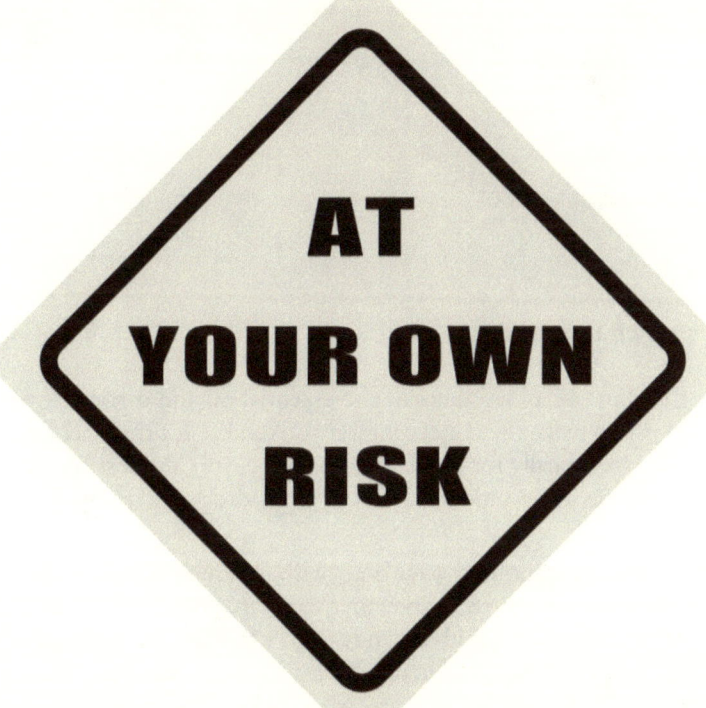

It is widely considered that **essential oils cannot cause or trigger your allergies**, as shown by this statement from Ever Faith:

"Because of the nature of distillation by heat, steam, and water, that true essential oils must undergo, they do not contain the necessary compounds to trigger allergies because these compounds do not pass through the distillation process. Hence, sensitivities to essential oils, in the sense of allergic reactions, are not possible. Allergic sensitivities are due to the body

developing antibodies in response to certain nitrogenous molecules. No one has ever found antibodies in humans from essential oils. So if one has a reaction to an essential oil, it is something else. Not an allergy."

Every person's body chemistry is different, though, and each will react in its own way to essential oils. Which is why we advise, no matter what your condition is: **you should always do a patch test before using any oil**. Doing so will allow you to know more accurately which oils are most appropriate for you.

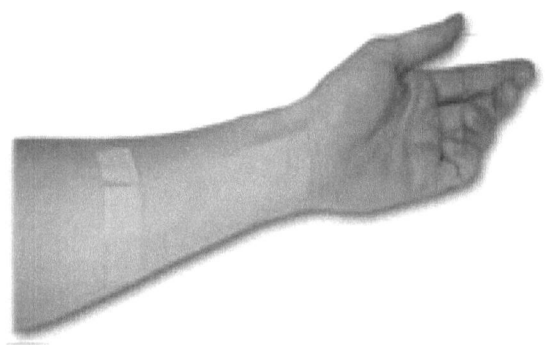

Here is a **patch test guide**:

1. Combine small amounts of the essential oil and carrier oil you plan to use to twice the concentration you require for treatment. Let's say your blend calls for a 3% concentration, mix the test blend for 6% (base this on a ratio of 3 essential oil drops for every 1/2 tsp. of carrier oil).

2. Choose a location on your body with minimal friction or direct sunlight exposure, such as the inner forearm, and cover the application of your test blend with a bandage. Try to keep the bandage in place for at least 48 hours. Then, look for signs of irritation.

3. Recreate the process to see if there will be any allergic reaction, but keep in mind that allergies may not develop right after initial exposure. So, just because there is no reaction now doesn't mean there won't ever be allergic reactions.

4. Skin reactions may include blisters, swelling, redness, or itchiness, and these will appear around or under the bandage. If this happens, avoid any future exposure to the tested essential oil.

You need to ensure that you **follow all of the instructions on how to use**

oils, and these Safety Tips to ensure that you get the best results from this treatment. It is also very advisable to read all of the ingredients in a product – for example, some products contain almonds, which would be terrible for a nut allergy sufferer. It is *always* best to seek advice from a medical professional before using essential oils.

That being said, there are some **essential oils that are considered unsafe for young children.** Here is a guide:

- **Anise/Aniseed** *(Pimpinella anisum, Illicium verum)* - avoid using (all routes) on children under 5

- **Basil (lemon)** *(Ocimum x citriodorum)* - avoid topical use on children under 2

- **Benzoin** *(Styrax benzoin, Styrax paralleloneurus,* and *Styrax tonkinensis)* - avoid topical use on children under 2

- **Birch (sweet)** *(Betula lenta)* - avoid using (all routes) on children

- **Black Seed** *(Nigella sativa)* - avoid topical use on children under 2

- **Cajeput** *(Melaleuca cajuputi, Melaleuca leucadendron)* - avoid using on children under 6

- **Cardamom** *(Elettaria cardamomum)* - avoid using (all routes) on children under 6

- **Cassia** *(Cinnamomum cassia, Cinnamomum aromaticum)* - avoid topical use on children under 2

- **Chaste Tree** *(Vitex agnus castus)* - avoid using (all routes) on prepubertal children

- **Clove Bud, Clove Leaf, Clove Stem** *(Syzygium aromaticum, Eugenia caryophyllata, Eugenia aromatica)* - avoid topical use on children under 2

- **Cornmint** *(Mentha arvensis, Mentha canadensis)* - avoid using (all routes) on children under 6

- **Eucalyptus** *(Eucalyptus camaldulensis, Eucalyptus globulus, Eucalyptus maidenii, Eucalyptus plenissima, Eucalyptus kochii, Eucalyptus polybractea, Eucalyptus radiata, Eucalyptus Autraliana, Eucalyptus phellandra, Eucalyptus smithii)* - avoid using (all routes) on children under 10

- **Fennel (bitter), Fennel (sweet)** *(Foeniculum vulgare)* - avoid using (all routes) on children under 5

- **Galangal (lesser)** *(Alpinia officinarum, Languas officinarum)* - avoid using (all routes) on children under 6

- **Garlic** (*Allium sativum*) - avoid topical use on children under 2

- **Ginger Lily** (*Hedychium coronarium*) - avoid topical use on children under 2

- **Ho Leaf/Ravensara** (*Cinnamomum camphora*) - avoid using on children under 6

- **Hyssop** (*Hyssopus officinalis*) - avoid using (all routes) on children under 2

- **Laurel Leaf/Bay Laurel** (*Laurus nobilis*) - avoid topical use on children under 2; avoid all routes for children under age 6

- **Lemon Leaf** (*Citrus x limon, Citrus limonum*) - avoid topical use on children under 2

- **Lemongrass** (*Cymbopogon flexuosus, Andropogon flexuosus, Cymbopogon citratus, Andropogon citratus*) - avoid topical use on children under 2

- **Marjoram** (*Thymus mastichina*) - avoid using (all routes) on children under 6

- **Massoia** (*Cryptocarya massoy, Cryptocaria massoia, Massoia aromatica*) - avoid using (all routes) on children under 2

- **May Chang** (*Litsea cubeba, Litsea citrata, Laura cubeba*) - avoid topical use on children under 2

- **Melissa/Lemon Balm** (*Melissa officinalis*) - avoid topical use on children under 2

- **Myrtle (red)** (*Myrtus communis*) - avoid using (all routes) on children under 6

- **Myrtle (aniseed)** (*Backhousia anisata*) - avoid using (all routes) on children under 5

- **Myrtle (honey)** (*Melaleuca teretifolia*) - avoid topical use on children under 2

- **Myrtle (lemon)/Sweet Verbena** (*Backhousia citriodora*) - avoid topical use on children under 2

- **Niaouli** (*Melaleuca quinquinervia*) - avoid using (all routes) on children under 6

- **Oakmoss** (*Evernia prunastri*) - avoid topical use on children under 2

- **Opopanax** (*Commiphora guidottii*) - avoid topical use on children under 2

- **Oregano** (*Origanum onites, Origanum smyrnaeum, Origanum vulgare, Origanum compactum, Origanum hirtum, Thymbra capitata, Thymus capitatus,*

Coridothymus capitatus, Satureeja capitata) - avoid topical use on children under 2

- **Peppermint** *(Mentha x Piperita)* - avoid using (all routes) on children under 6

- **Peru Balsam** *(Myroxylon balsamum, Myroxylon pereiraw, Myroxylon peruiferum, Myrospermum pereirae, Toluifera pereirae)* - avoid topical use on children under 2

- **Rambiazana** *(Helichrysum gymnocephalum)* - avoid using (all routes) on children under 6

- **Rosemary** *(Rosmarinus officinalis)* - avoid using (all routes) on children under 6

- **Saffron** *(Crocus sativus)* - avoid topical use on children under 2

- **Sage (Greek)** *(Salvia fruiticosa, Salvia triloba)* - avoid using (all routes) on children under 6

- **Sage (white)** *(Salvia apiana)* - avoid using (all routes) on children under 6

- **Sage (wild mountain)** *(Hemizygia petiolata)* - avoid topical use on children under 2

- **Sanna** *(Hedychium spicatum)* - avoid using (all routes) on children under 6

- **Saro** *(Cinnamosma fragrans)* - avoid using (all routes) on children under 6

- **Savory** *(Satureia hortensis, Satureia Montana)* - avoid topical use on children under 2

- **Styrax** *(Liquidambar orientalis, Liquidambar styraciflua)* - avoid topical use on children under 2

- **Tea Leaf/Black Tea** *(Camellia sinensis, Thea sinensis)* - avoid topical use on children under 2

- **Tea Tree (lemon scented)** *(Leptospermum petersonii, Leptospermum citratum, Leptospermum liversidgei)* - avoid topical use on children under 2

- **Treemoss** *(Pseudevernia furfuracea)* - avoid topical use on children under 2

- **Tuberose** *(Polianthes tuberose)* - avoid topical use on children under 2

- **Turpentine** *(Pinus ayacahuite, Pinus caribaea, Pinus contorta, Pinus elliottii, Pinus halepensis, Pinus insularis, Pinus kesiya, Pinus merkusii, Pinus palustris, Pinus pinaster, Pinus radiata, Pinus roxburghii, Pinus tabulaeformis,*

Pinus teocote, Pinus yunnanensis) - avoid topical use on children under 2

- **Verbena (lemon)** (*Aloysia triphylla, Aloysia citriodora, Lippa citriodora, Lippa triphylla*) - avoid topical use on children under 2

- **Wintergreen** (*Gaultheria fragrantissima, Gaultheria procumbens*) – avoid (all routes) on children due to methyl salicylate content

- **Ylang Ylang** (*Cananga odorata*) - avoid topical use on children under 2.

For more information on how to use these essential oils with your children, refer to the "Dilution" chapter of this book.

There are also some scenarios in which you should **avoid certain essential oils as an adult** – for example, if you're pregnant, elderly, or suffering from certain health conditions. A lot of these are covered in the "Safety" chapter of this book.

For extra information on this topic, there are many online resources such as:

Wellness Mama *at wellnessmama.com/26519/risks-essential-oil*

Taking Charge *at www.takingcharge.csh.umn.edu*

But of course, it is always advisable to speak to a health professional before using any of the products – especially if you have any concerns.

50 LITTLE KNOWN ESSENTIAL OIL RECIPES

This chapter is going to give you some recipes for common ailments that you can create in your own kitchen. Just remember all of the dilution and blending rules as you follow the instructions below.

1. Homemade Cellulite Massage Oil

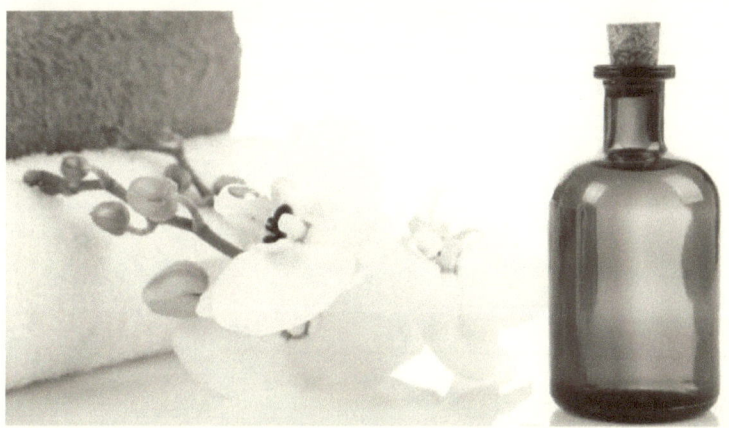

Unwanted cellulite can cause a lot of issues for people, and this oil is designed to combat it. This blend is for adult usage, and is to be applied topically to the affected area.

Ingredients:

- 1/4 cup of Sweet Almond oil
- 1/4 cup of Jojoba oil

- 10 drops each of Juniper, Cinnamon Leaf, Orange, and Cypress essential oils

Directions:

- Pour the directed amount of each into a bottle with a cap.
- Cap it up and shake thoroughly before using.

2. Headache Eraser

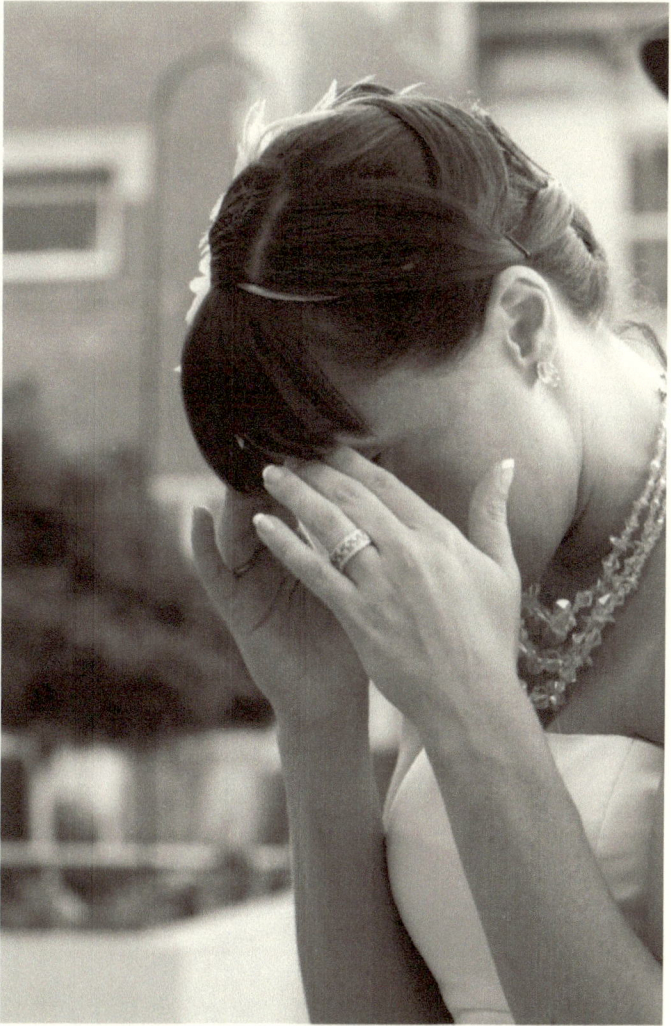

Headaches can really affect the way you feel, the way you act, and what you can do. This recipe is designed for adult usage, and can be diluted for your needs. The blend is to be applied topically to the affected area.

Ingredients:

- 10-20 drops each of Eucalyptus, Cajeput, Lavender, Peppermint, and Rosemary essential oils

- 5 drops of Roman Chamomile essential oil (optional)
- 1 drop of Helichrysum essential oil (optional)
- 2-3 mL of Carrier oil (such as Safflower or Grapeseed) or Perfumery alcohol

Directions:

- Find a 5 mL glass or roll-on bottle.
- Start by adding your preferred blend of the suggested oils.
- Fill the bottle's remaining space with the carrier oil or perfumery alcohol that you prefer. Note: the alcohol will evaporate faster than the oil will.

3. Addiction First Aid Kit

Addiction can have a massive impact on your everyday life. Select your ailment from the list below and blend the essential oils appropriately. Be sure to perform a patch test and dilute as necessary.

Behavior

- **Anxiety**: Lavender and Ylang Ylang
- **Cravings**: Cilantro, Cinnamon, Clove, Grapefruit, and Peppermint
- **Eating Disorders**: Bergamot, Cinnamon, and Grapefruit
- **Porn**: Frankincense
- **Sex**: Geranium and Sandalwood
- **Withdrawal**: Grapefruit, Lavender, Orange (and other citrus), Marjoram, and Sandalwood
- **Work addiction**: Basil, Lavender, Orange, and Ylang Ylang

Substances

- **Alcohol**: Basil, Chamomile, Frankincense, and Rosemary
- **Caffeine**: Grapefruit and Basil
- **Drugs**: Basil, Chamomile, and Grapefruit
- **Food**: Basil and Grapefruit
- **Sugar**: Bergamot and Grapefruit
- **Tobacco**: Basil, Black Pepper, and Clove

4. Anti-Inflammatory Foot Oil

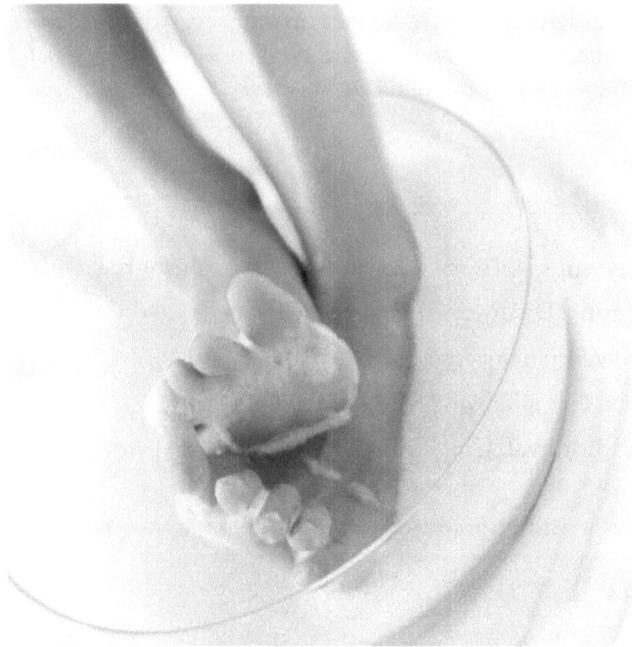

Our feet go through so much on a daily basis and having them out of action can be a nightmare! Use this antimicrobial blend by massaging onto cracked, itchy, peeling, and irritated skin. This blend is strong enough for adults and can be applied directly to the area of concern.

Ingredients:

- Tea Tree essential oil – 6 drops
- Lavender essential oil – 4 drops
- Chamomile essential oil – 6 drops
- 30-35 mL of Carrier oil (such as Olive or Coconut)

Directions:

Find a dark glass bottle. Blend equal parts Tea Tree and Chamomile oils with Lavender, using 2 drops less than amount of other oils, and carrier oil of your choice. Pour mixture into the bottle. Use this blend before going to bed or even putting on socks for the day.

5. Blend For Arthritis Joint Care

Pain is an awful part of everyday life with arthritis, and this blend is designed to help you with that. It's for adult usage, can be diluted to suit, and is to be applied topically to the affected area.

Ingredients:

- Peppermint essential oil
- Ginger essential oil
- Black Pepper essential oil
- Juniper Berry essential oil
- Eucalyptus Globulus essential oil
- V-6 carrier oil

Directions:

Find a 4 oz. bottle. Add up to 20 drops of each essential oil to the bottle. Fill remaining space in the bottle with the carrier oil. Be sure to mix well.

Note: You will use only a small amount, due to its being almost 5% concentration of oil. Be sure to patch test first; there will be a strong warming effect. This blend works better in a specific area of concern versus use for a whole back or body massage. For example, focus use on your shoulders, neck, or down spinal column.

6. Soothing Blend For Menstrual Cramps

Menstrual cramps are an issue for most women – but for some, this pain can be debilitating – monthly! Below is a great blend to be used topically, for adults.

Ingredients:

- 3/4 cup of Olive oil or Coconut oil
- 1/4 cup of Beeswax, pebbles or grated
- 30 drops of Geranium essential oil
- 40 drops of Lavender essential oil
- 25 drops of Roman Chamomile essential oil
- 25 drops of Clary Sage essential oil
- 30 drops of Bergamot essential oil
- 40 drops of Ginger essential oil
- 60 drops of Clove essential oil
- 1/2 tsp. of Vitamin E (optional)

Directions:

- Put a small pan over medium heat with an inch of water at the bottom. Without getting water inside, set a glass jar (holding a pint or two) inside the pan. Add beeswax and Olive or Coconut oil, then completely melt.
- After those ingredients have melted and been thoroughly combined, take off of the heat. When mixture has cooled, stir in remaining oils and Vitamin E.
- Before use, allow blend to cool and harden. This recipe will yield approximately 1 cup (or 8 oz.). Store blend in shallow, round tins.

7. Labor

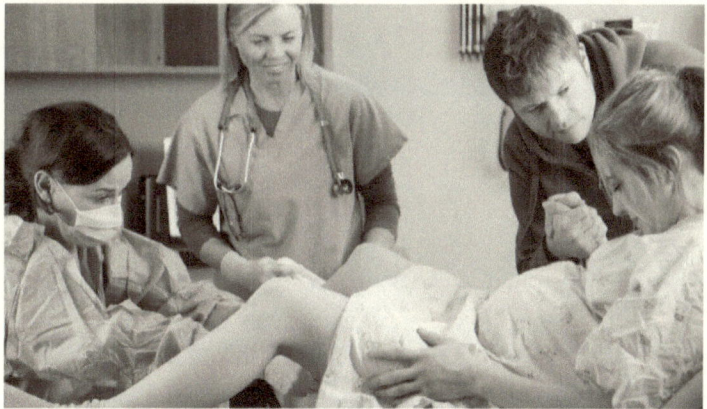

There isn't much that can help with childbirth, but below is a recipe for top-ical use to help ease the pain in a natural way. This can be diluted to suit if necessary.

Ingredients:

- 4 drops of Helichrysum essential oil
- 4 drops of Fennel essential oil
- 2 drops of Peppermint essential oil
- 5 drops of Ylang Ylang essential oil
- 3 drops of Clary Sage essential oil
- 1/2 oz. V-6 carrier oil

Directions:

Wait until labor starts, then massage her lower tummy and back, little fingers and toes, and inside her ankles.

Alternatively, the following **diffusing blend** can be used during labor:

- 40 drops of Lavender essential oil
- 37 drops of Frankincense essential oil
- 21 drops of Ylang Ylang essential oil
- 20 drops of Roman Chamomile essential oil

8. Weight Loss Blends

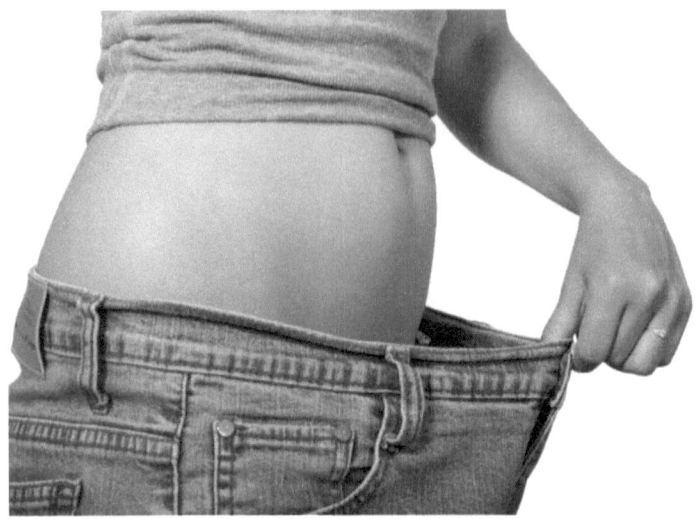

Losing weight can be challenging. Many essential oil users claim that they make the process much more bearable. An essential oil that is the most famous for assisting in weight loss is Grapefruit essential oil.

These three blends below, for adult usage, may provide effective assistance. Use the "Dilution" chapter of this book if you wish to change the recipe to suit your personal needs.

Citrus Blend Ingredients:

- 30 drops of Grapefruit essential oil
- 4 drops of Lemon essential oil
- 1 drop of Ylang Ylang essential oil

Mint Blend Ingredients:

- 20 drops of Peppermint essential oil
- 10 drops of Bergamot essential oil
- 4 drops of Spearmint essential oil
- 1 drop of Ylang Ylang essential oil

Herbal Blend Ingredients:

- 15 drops of Basil essential oil
- 15 drops of Marjoram essential oil
- 1 drop of Oregano essential oil
- 1 drop of Thyme essential oil

Directions:

Find a small, dark glass bottle. Start with 1 tsp. of coarse sea salt at the bottom of the bottle, then add one of the suggested blends.

To use: draw 3 slow, deep breaths from the bottle. Pause for a moment before taking 3 more slow, deep breaths. Only take this series of breaths 3 times.

This inhaler is portable, and can be used anywhere before eating or whenever you feel hungry. Studies have shown that when you inhale essential oils more often, they will be more effective. There are even studies that suggest aromatherapy can be even more effective toward weight loss when you regularly alternate between scents. This is why we have provided you with multiple blends to make. Select one blend that will be used on Monday, Wednesday, and Saturday; another could be used on Tuesday and Thursday, and the third could be used on Sunday, for example. Feel free to personalize this arrangement to suit your needs.

9. Hangover Cure

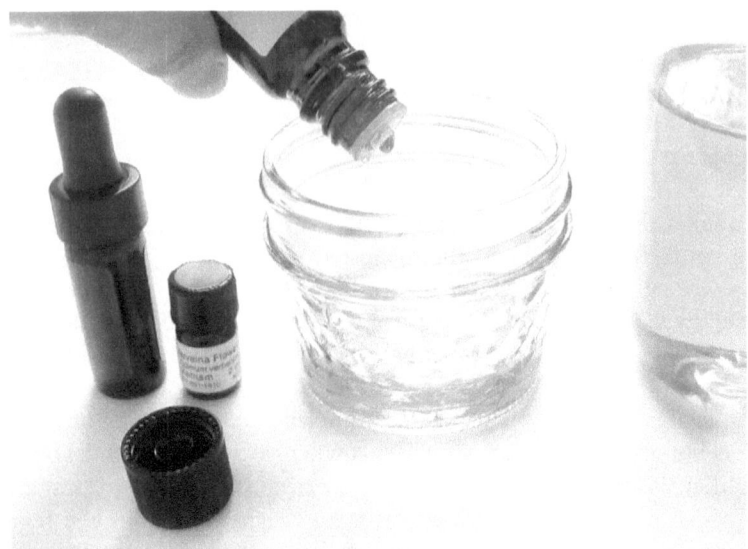

We've all been there at some point – had just one too many. This blend is a detox for those hangover days. Of course, it's for adult usage, to be applied topically, and can be diluted to your personal requirements.

Ingredients:

- 15 drops of Peppermint essential oil
- 10 drops of Lavender essential oil
- 1 oz. pure Water

Directions:

Combine the ingredients well and dab them on the back of your neck and your wrists to rid your body of the awful hangover.

10. Anti-Aging Facial Serum

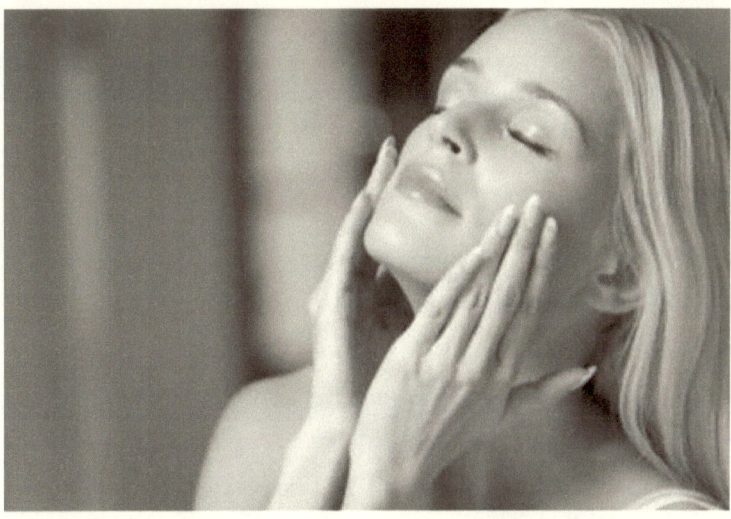

The wrinkle cream industry is massive. This recipe has been designed so you can create your own effective oil, saving you money! It's for adult usage and is to be applied topically and can be diluted to your preference. This mixture would make a great nightly serum for your face.

Ingredients:

- 1/2 cup of Apricot Kernel oil
- 10 drops (not shakes) of Carrot Seed essential oil
- 10 drops of Rosehip Seed essential oil

Directions:

- Combine and keep in amber bottle.
- Rub a small amount into cleansed face and neck.

11. Homemade Shampoo

As more and more people turn to natural treatments, essential oil shampoo is becoming increasingly popular. Below is a list of great smelling, useful combinations for you to create your very own personalized hair care product. These recipes are recommended for adult use only:

Ingredients:

- 3/4 cup of liquid Castile Soap
- 1/2 cup of canned Coconut Milk
- 1/2 cup of Honey
- 3 tbsp. of fractionated Coconut oil
- 2 tbsp. of Vitamin E oil
- Up to 60-70 drops of essential oils (select from options below)
  - 30 drops of Lavender and 35-40 drops of Wild Orange essential oils
  - 40 drops of Lavender and 30 drops of Peppermint essential oils (if you prefer, substitute Wild Orange for Lavender)
  - 20 drops of Lavender, 15 drops of Lemon, and 30 drops of Lemongrass essential oils
  - *Treating fragile hair:* 20 drops of Lavender, 25 drops of Clary Sage, and 20 drops of Wild Orange essential oils
  - *Treating hair loss:* Lavender, Rosemary, Cedarwood, and Peppermint essential oils (20 drops of each)
  - *Treating dandruff:* Lavender, Rosemary, Lemon, and Tea Tree essential oils (20 drops of each)

Directions:

Find a squeeze bottle. Combine the ingredients in the bottle. Close the bottle's lid tightly and shake. Use like any commercial shampoo. Remember to shake before every use.

12. Baby Massage Oil

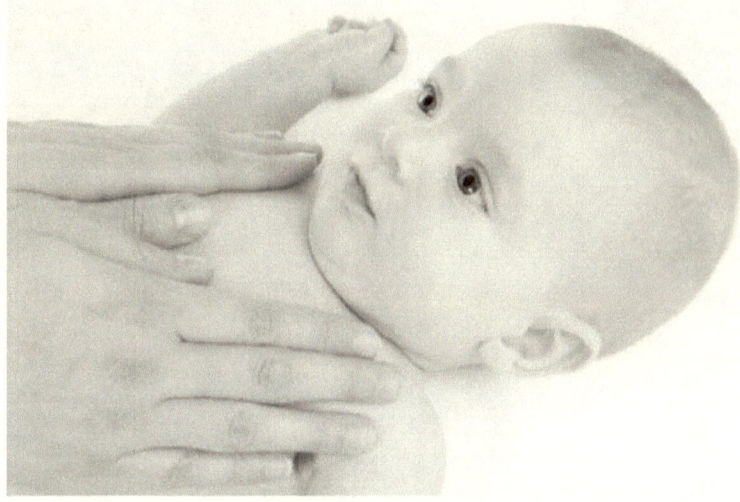

Baby massage is very popular, and for good reason! It can help babies sleep, ease colic and other stomach issues, and is very relaxing for mother and baby. This blend will help you to do this from home.

Ingredients:

- 1 drop of Lavender essential oil or Chamomile essential oil
- 2 tbsp. of Sweet Almond carrier oil

Directions:

- Add essential oil to sweet almond oil and blend.
- Apply this mixture topically while giving your baby a relaxing massage.
- Increase essential oils to up to 5 drops for every 2 tbsp. of carrier oil after your baby is more than two months old.

Treating **diaper rash** – mix 1 drop of Lavender and 1 drop of German Chamomile essential oils with 1 pint of warm water. Store in a clean jar. Apply this blend by dipping a cotton ball into it, then wiping directly on the area of concern.

13. Anxiety Bath Blend

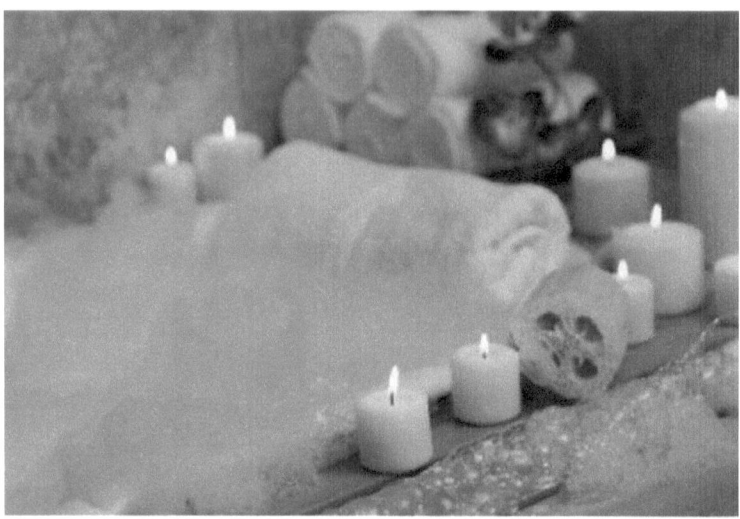

Anxiety, stress, and depression are terrifying parts of everyday life. Increasing numbers of people are suffering from them. There is a recipe for adults, to be taken aromatically in a bath, to assist sufferers with this. This blend can be adjusted to suit your preferences, so you can select an oil from the list below for this. The "Dilution" chapter of this book can give you some good advice on how ensure the recipe suits your skin.

Ingredients:

- *Bergamot* – an uplifting scent that helps with feelings of pain, anxiety, and depression.

- *Basil* – a refreshing scent that works against anxiety, depression, and fatigue.

- *Clary Sage* – helps eradicate feelings of anxiety, depression, and insomnia.

- *Frankincense* – helps alleviate feelings of anxiety, stress, and nervous tension.

- *Geranium* – a natural sedative that uplifts your spirit by releasing negative emotions; eases the symptoms of stress and depression.

- *Jasmine* – a relaxing flowery scent known to be an antispasmodic.

- *Lemon* – a refreshing scent with purifying, uplifting properties; boosts immunity and helps ease the negative emotions of stress and depression.

- *Lavender* – considered a cure-all; helps ease migraine and headache, anxiety and fear, depression and insomnia, nervousness, and hypertension; provides a calming and relaxing effect for both mind and body.

- *Mandarin* – works to lift the spirit and offers antispasmodic properties.

- *Marjoram* – eases the feelings of rejection, anxiety and fear, grief and loneliness.

- *Wild Orange* – provides an energizing, mood-lifting, and refreshing effect; works to ease feelings of irritation, panic, nervousness, and anger.

- *Palmarosa* – helps to ease anxiety and nervous tension.

- *Rose* – a stimulating aroma that creates a sense of well-being, having an effect on your whole nervous system.

- *Roman Chamomile* – relaxes and calms both mind and body; has been used in easing stress and depression.

- *Sandalwood* – a comforting aroma with sedative properties; eases inner stress and tension.

- *Ylang Ylang* – a relaxing scent; known to bring balance to the spirit's female and male energies; has been used to restore equilibrium and confidence and treat anxiety, insomnia, and depression.

Directions:

Gently mix up to 10 drops of the essential oils into your bathwater after you have finished running it. Adding them to running water will make them evaporate more quickly. Dilute the oils, before adding them to the water, with up to 1 tbsp. of your preferred carrier oil if you have sensitive skin. Use a personalized blend from among the oils listed above to alleviate anxious, stressed, or depressed feelings.

14. Under The Weather Blend For Children

It's very difficult for children when they are under the weather. This blend has been designed to combat that – it is to be used aromatically, in a bath.

Ingredients:

- 2 drops of Manuka essential oil
- 2 drops of Eucalyptus Radiata essential oil
- 2 drops of Lavender essential oil
- 1 cup of Epsom Salts

Directions:

- Combine essential oils with salts, mixing well.
- Pour salt blend into running bathwater. Make swirling motions in water to blend into the water.
- Soak for up to 20 minutes.

This blend is for a 10-year-old but can be diluted according to the child's age.

15. An Energy Boost

Tiredness and fatigue can really ruin your day. This blend can be mixed for a needed boost. Many essential oil users swear by this recipe, which is for adult usage and to be used aromatically. If you need to change this blend to suit your personalized needs, use the "Dilution" chapter of this book.

Ingredients:

- 2 drops of Wild Orange essential oil
- 2 drops of Peppermint essential oil

Directions:

- In the palm of one hand, add the Peppermint oil first, then add the Wild Orange oil. Rub the palms of both of your hands together.
- Make a fist with one hand, while holding the other flat and facing your mouth. Place the bottom of your fist on top of your palm. Lightly press your mouth against your fist and inhale deeply, so you take the aromas in through your fist.

16. Vapor Balm

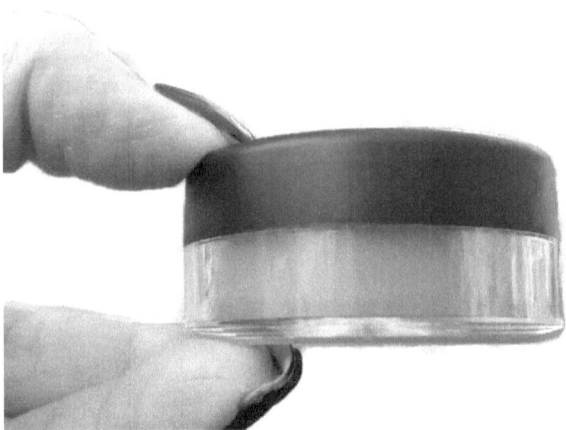

For any issues with your respiratory system, there is an essential oil blend for adult use to be used aromatically – as a burner/candle. You can use the "Dilution" chapter of this book to edit the recipe if necessary.

Ingredients:

- 2 tsp. of Peppermint essential oil
- 3 tsp. of Eucalyptus essential oil
- 1 tsp. of Thyme essential oil (chemotype linalool is best)
- 1 cup of Olive oil
- 3/4 oz. of Beeswax

Directions:

Over low heat, melt the beeswax and Olive oil. Let this mixture cool. Add essential oils to mixture, then stir. Note: keep your face turned away from the oils while you stir. Store at room temperature after the blend hardens.

17. After Sun

Sunburn is nasty and painful. Calming the redness and soothing the pain through essential oils with this recipe is a great way to do get rid of it naturally. The blend is to be used topically, for adults, and can be changed to suit using the "Dilution" chapter of this book.

Ingredients:

- 1/2 cup of Witch Hazel
- 2 tbsp. of pure Aloe Vera gel
- 10 drops of pure Lavender essential oil
- 10 drops of pure Peppermint essential oil
- 4 oz. (or larger) spray bottle

Directions:

- In a small mixing bowl with a spout, combine the ingredients by mixing well. Pour the blend into your spray bottle, then shake well. This can be applied generously to the area of concern. Note: avoid spraying into or around your eyes, there will be a stinging sensation.
- The blend will feel sticky at first, but that goes away as it dries on the skin.
- Reapply every 30 minutes at first, then as needed.

18. Handmade Eczema Cream

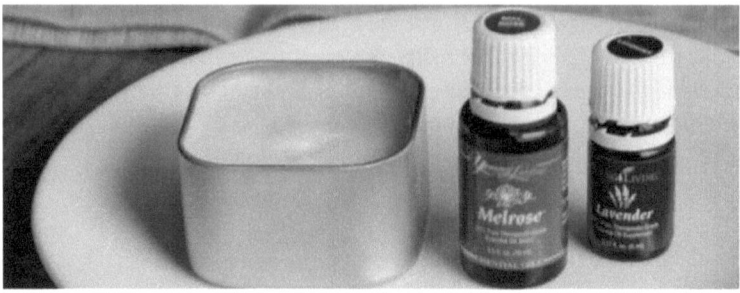

This recipe is great for sensitive skin and is to be applied topically to the affected area. It's suitable for all ages, including babies.

Ingredients:

- 1/4 cup of Coconut oil (soft or melted)
- 1/4 cup of Shea Butter
- 1/2 tsp. of Vitamin E oil
- 25 drops of Melrose essential oil
- 15 drops of Lavender essential oil

Directions:

- Find a 4 oz. or larger container to store finished product. Using a small bowl, whisk or stir Vitamin E oil, shea butter, and Coconut oil well.
- Add the essential oils, stirring until they are well incorporated.
- Transfer mixed cream to your preferred container. It is best to store at room temperature; if you keep your home warm (more than 75 degrees) the cream can lose some of its consistency. If this bothers you, feel free to store in the fridge.
- These proportions will produce nearly 4 oz. of cream. It's for topical application on the affected area.

19. Rash

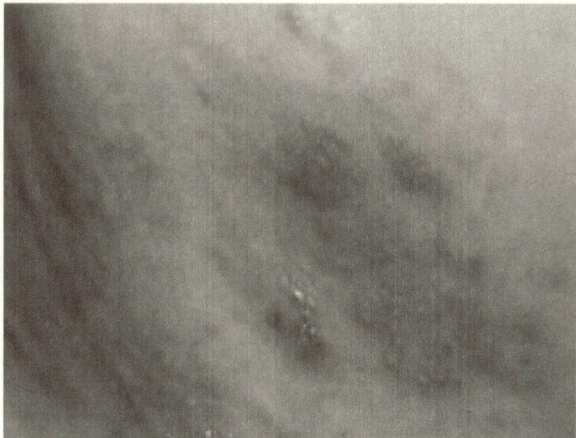

Here are a few essential oil treatments for rashes. They can be used for any age but be careful with very young children. Refer to the "Dilution" chapter of the book for more information. This blend is to be used aromatically in a bath.

Ingredients:

- Lavender essential oil
- Chamomile essential oil
- Eucalyptus essential oil

Directions:

Add each essential oil to warm bathwater, just a few drops. You don't need to use them all. If you only have one, feel free to use it solo. Soak for about 20 minutes.

Serum

Ingredients:

- Baking Soda
- Lavender essential oil

Directions:

Blend baking soda with essential oil, alternating the soda with a few drops of oil. Apply blend directly to area of concern, cover completely.

This heat rash serum could be used on babies or infants. Note: make sure baby's skin, especially the folds, is totally dry. When treating infants, under 2 years of age, reduce to 1/4 cup of soda and 2-3 drops of the oil. When treating babies and older children (between 2-12 years), increase soda and oil proportionately after a patch test to determine skin sensitivity. When treating adults, mix about 1 cup of soda with up to 8 drops of oil.

20. Digestive Blend

Any sort of stomach pain can impact your health massively. Below is a list of the best oils to use in your diffuser to help with this (adult use only):

- *Peppermint*: Works as a pain reliever, has anti-inflammatory properties, and eases stomach cramps and aches.

- *Tarragon*: Curbs gas dyspepsia, nervous digestion, and even urinary tract infections (UTI).

- *Ginger*: In addition to calming the digestive system, it also bolsters emotional well-being. It is known for having other properties such as tonic, antiseptic, stimulant, and laxative. Ginger is often used for nausea, vomiting, diarrhea, and motion sickness.

- *Fennel*: Often used for gastritis, parasites, kidney stones, cleansing the toxins, and other matters pertaining to digestive support.

- *Coriander*: Used for helping gas, diarrhea, and indigestion. Known for being antibacterial, analgesic, antifungal, and anti-inflammatory.

- *Caraway*: Antispasmodic and antiparasitic, Caraway assists with gas, indigestion, and digestive tract spasms.

- *Anise*: Helps in calming and strengthening the digestive system.

21. Muscle Spasm Blend

This blend has been designed to help ease the pain of cramping and spasming muscles by helping them to relax. It is to be applied topically to the affected area, for adult use, and can be adjusted according to your personal requirements using the "Dilution" chapter of this book.

Ingredients:

- 20 drops of Basil essential oil
- 15 drops of Marjoram essential oil
- 15 drops of Lemongrass essential oil
- 5 drops of Frankincense essential oil
- fractionated Coconut oil

Directions:

- Put essential oils into roll-on bottle and fill remainder of bottle with fractionated Coconut oil.
- Roll on oil blend as needed.

22. Bad Breath Blend

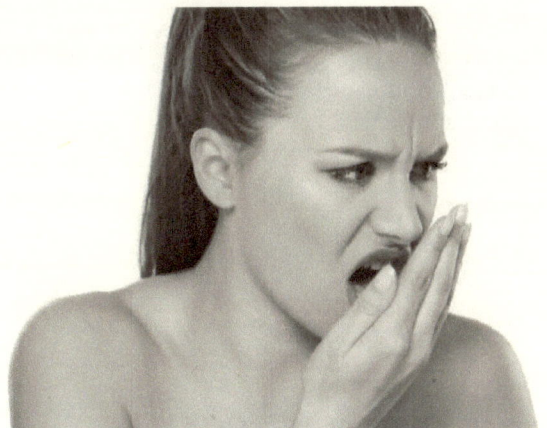

There can be many causes of bad breath, and below is a selection of recipes to help with any of them. It's for adult use only and is to be applied topically.

Bad Breath Due to Digestive Issues:

- 2 drops of Peppermint essential oil
- 2 drops of Lemon essential oil

Bad Breath Due to Gum Disease:

- 2 drops of Tea Tree essential oil
- 2 drops of Thyme essential oil

General:

- 4 drops of Lavender essential oil

Directions:

For each recipe, dilute the essential oil in 1 tsp. of brandy and add to a tumbler of warm water. Take a sip, rinse around your mouth, and spit out. Make sure you do not swallow any of the liquid.

23. Hives Skin Wash

Hives are the red, itchy patches of skin that appear as a result of allergies. Here is a blend for using essential oils to get rid of hives. This recipe is for adult usage but can be adjusted to suit your needs via the "Dilution" chapter of this book and is for topical application.

Ingredients:

- 5 drops of Chamomile essential oil or 10 drops of Lavender essential oil
- 2 drops of Peppermint essential oil
- 3 tbsp. of Baking Soda
- 2 cups of Water (or use Peppermint Tea instead)

Directions:

Combine the ingredients. If you are making a tea to use as the base instead of water, pour 2 1/2 cups of boiling water over 4 tsp. of dried peppermint leaves and steep 15 minutes. Strain out the herb. Add the remaining ingredients. Use a soft cloth or a skin sponge to apply on irritated skin until itching is alleviated. Chamomile is the best choice for this recipe, but it is expensive, so 10 drops of Lavender essential oil can be substituted, if necessary.

24. Lip Chap

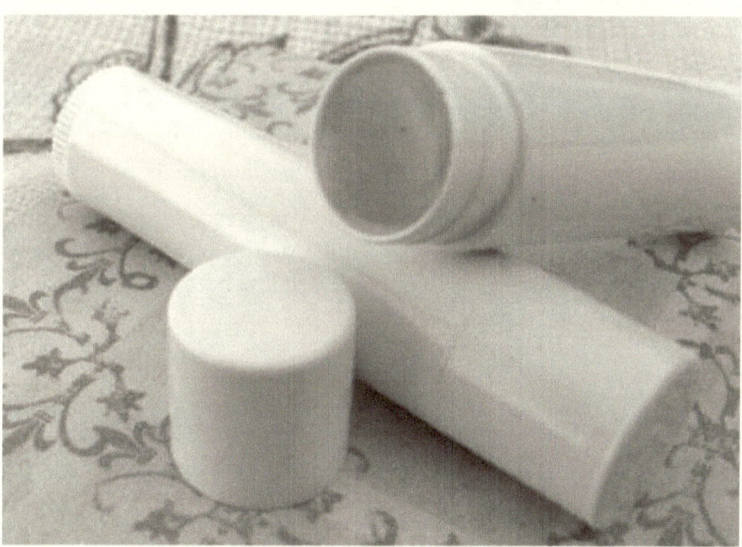

This lip balm is a brilliant and easy recipe that you can create at home. It is for adult usage and is to be applied topically.

Ingredients:

- 1 tbsp. of Beeswax
- 2 tbsp. of Shea, Cocoa, or Mango Butter
- 2 tbsp. of Coconut oil
- 20 drops of Peppermint essential oil

Directions:

- Put a small pan over medium heat with an inch of water at the bottom. Without getting water inside, set a glass jar (pint or smaller) inside the pan.
- Except essential oil, slowly melt all ingredients in the glass jar. Proportions of beeswax and butters above can fill almost 18 lip chap tubes.
- After those ingredients have melted, stir well then turn off heat from under pan. You want to keep the jar warm, though, so keep it in the water.

- Slowly mix in essential oil with melted ingredients in the jar. A glass dropper can be used to fill lip chap tubes. Leaving the jar in the water will help ingredients maintain liquid state.

- As the mixture cools, it will settle. Add a bit more of the melted ingredients from the jar to top off the tubes. Wait for the mix to start to harden, just a couple minutes. The mixture should be fully settled after several hours. Store tubes in a dry, cool space.

- These proportions and directions will create a medium firm consistency. Use more beeswax for a firmer consistency, but no more than twice the amount suggested. Use less beeswax for an oilier consistency.

25. Stop Snoring

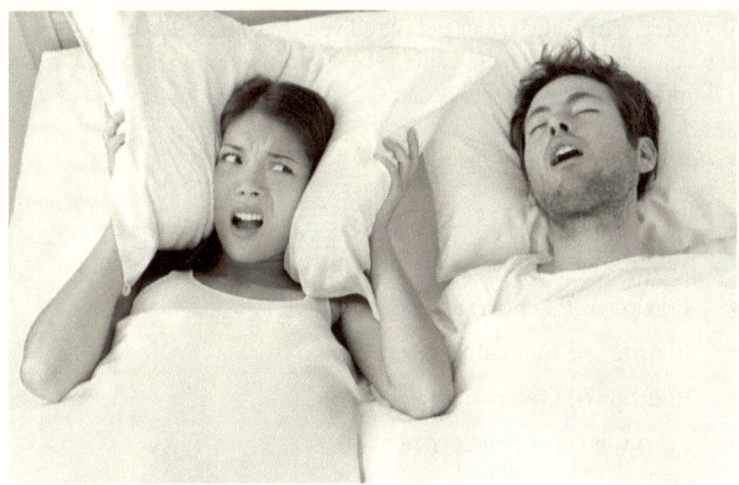

Snoring can lead to a vicious cycle. It leads to less sleep, and if you are exhausted, your snoring can get worse. This recipe is great for snoring. It's for adult usage, to be applied topically, and can be diluted to suit. Note: use Thyme in a humidifier to ease restless sleep.

Ingredients:

- 4-6 drops of undiluted Thyme essential oil
- 4-6 drops of Carrier oil (a vegetable oil you prefer)

Directions:

Dilute the Thyme with your preferred carrier oil. Rub on the bottom of your feet before you go to bed.

26. Psoriasis Recipe

Skin disorders can really affect people's lives. This psoriasis blend is for adult usage, to be applied topically. This recipe can be changed to suit you using the "Dilution" chapter of this book.

Ingredients:

- 6 tbsp. of Carrier oil (such as Sweet Almond oil, Avocado oil, Coconut oil, Pumpkin Seed oil, Rosehip Seed oil, Kukui Nut oil, etc.)
- 4 drops of Patchouli essential oil
- 10 drops of Frankincense essential oil
- 10 drops of Geranium essential oil
- 1 drop of Clary Sage essential oil
- 11 drops of Lavender essential oil
- 3 drops of Mandarin essential oil
- 1 drop of Ylang Ylang essential oil
- 9 drops of Bergamot essential oil

Directions:

- Find a dark glass dropper bottle. Add your preferred carrier oil, then the essential oils. Note: Be aware of the grade of the essential oils. This will have an impact on the treatment's effectiveness. Try to use only the very best oils from a company you trust.
- Close the bottle tightly and shake gently to blend. Twice a day, use the amount of oil you need to treat your psoriasis.

27. Air Freshener

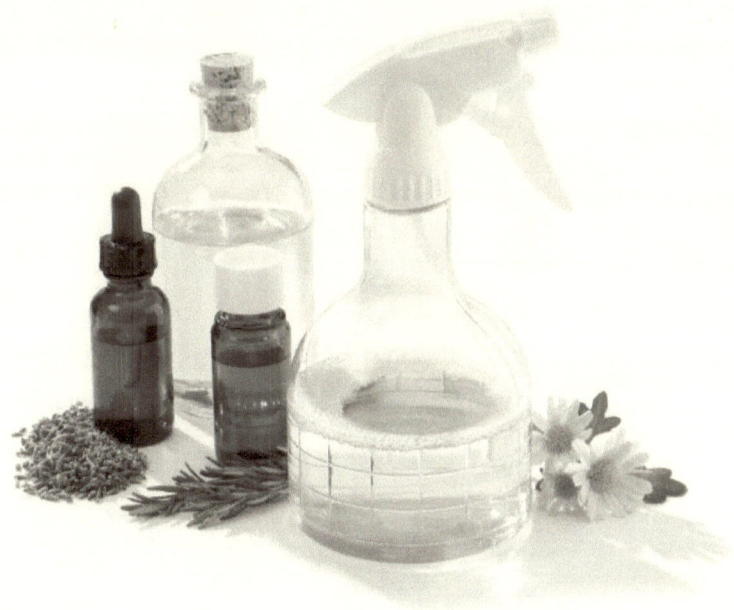

Did you know that essential oils can also be used around the home? This recipe is for an air freshener.

Ingredients:

- A clean, empty spray bottle
- 1 cup of Water
- 2 tbsp. of Vodka (unflavored and non-diluted)
- 20 drops* of Essential oil (choose one from the list below)
    - Lemon: reduces anxiety and works like an antidepressant
    - Orange: relaxes and rejuvenates
    - Clary Sage: can bring calm to your nervous system
    - Rosemary: can improve memory and invigorate the mind
    - Clove: works as an aphrodisiac and can bring relief to congested nasal passages
    - Lavender: can also bring calm to your nervous system and improve the quality of your sleep
    - Basil: reduces the pain of headaches

Directions:

- Start by adding the water to the spray bottle.
- Pour in essential oils (*start conservatively when adding oils, some are stronger and can overwhelm the blend), then vodka.
- Tightly close spray bottle, then shake to combine.

28. Pet Care

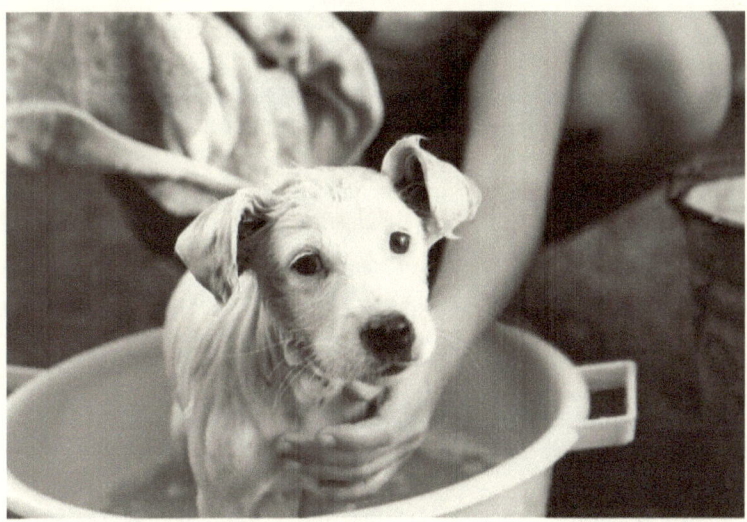

Essential oils can also be used in the care of your animals, as shown by this example recipe for dog shampoo. This can be helpful to support the skin and coat, building up your dog's immunity.

Ingredients:

- 1 cup of Water
- 1 tbsp. of Castile Soap
- 1/4 tsp. of Vitamin E
- 3 drops of Peppermint essential oil
- 3 drops of Lavender essential oil
- 2 drops of Roman Chamomile essential oil
- 2 drops of Purification essential oil blend
- 1 drop of Cedarwood essential oil
- 2 drops of Citronella (optional)

Directions:

Mix all of this together in a jar and use straight. This recipe is suitable for a dog of any age, but seek advice if your dog is very young, very old, or has sensitive skin. It's watery but use it like you would normal dog shampoo.

29. Sleepy Spray

Lack of sleep can be torturous and can impact nastily on your daily life. If you're having trouble, here is a great recipe for this. This recipe is suitable for adults and is to be used topically. Refer to the "Dilution" chapter of this book if you want to adjust this to suit you.

Ingredients:

- Almost 2 oz. of Ancient Minerals Magnesium oil.
- 20 drops of Peace&Calming essential oil blend, or Lavender, Cedarwood, or Roman Chamomile essential oils.
- 2 oz. dark glass spray bottle.

Directions:

Start by adding enough Ancient Minerals Magnesium oil to fill the spray bottle. Mix in the essential oils and blends. Tightly close the bottle, then shake well. Apply by massaging into the bottom of your feet about 20 minutes before you go to sleep. Then, you could cup your hands to inhale the oil remaining there for an extra benefit.

30. Bruise Blend

Unsightly bruises can be difficult to get rid of. This recipe can help you get rid of the pain and the bruise. It is for adult use, to be applied topically and can be diluted to suit.

Ingredients:

- 5 drops of Helichrysum essential oil
- 4 drops of Lavender essential oil
- 3 drops of Cypress essential oil
- 3 drops of Lemongrass essential oil
- 3 drops of Geranium essential oil

Directions:

Can your bruise be immediately tended to? Lavender and Cypress will constrict blood vessels and ease the pain. Anywhere within the first 6-24 hours, when the swelling has most likely stopped, constricting the blood vessels needs to be replaced with increasing circulation to the injury in order to heal the bruise more quickly. Do this by using up to 3 drops of the Helichrysum every couple hours. The complete blend above, though, can offer even more relief.

Note: the more quickly cold can be placed on the injury, the less likely bruising will occur. You can better protect your skin by applying the ice indirectly, alternating between hot and cold compresses, on the area. It is best not to continuously leave ice, or heat, on the injury. We recommend 15 minutes on and 15 minutes off for applying ice to the injury.

31. Depression Inhaler

This aromatherapy inhaler is great because it's portable; make a couple or one of each and keep one at your desk, in your bag, or in your car to use whenever it's needed. You can choose one of the blends listed below, depending on what suits you. They are for adult use, to be used aromatically, and can be diluted if necessary.

Mood Lifter for Irritable Depression Ingredients:

- 10 drops of Bergamot essential oil
- 5 drops of Grapefruit essential oil
- 4 drops of Sweet Orange essential oil
- 1 drop of Geranium essential oil
- 1 drop of Ylang Ylang essential oil

Comforting Blend for Grief-related Depression Ingredients:

- 10 drops of Rose Absolute essential oil or Rose Otto essential oil
- 4 drops of Sandalwood essential oil
- 4 drops of Neroli essential oil or Petitgrain essential oil

Soothing Blend for Anxious Depression Ingredients:

- 8 drops of Lavender essential oil
- 8 drops of Grapefruit essential oil
- 2 drops of Marjoram essential oil
- 1 drop of Chamomile essential oil
- 1 drop of Geranium essential oil

Directions:

- Find 1-3 dark, glass bottles. Add 1 tsp. of coarse sea salt to the bottom of each, then add an oil blend.
- Apply by taking 3 slow, deep breaths over the top of the bottle. When you really feel blue or frustrated, pause after those first 3 breaths, then take 3 more. Only take this application 3 times.
- After the scent begins to fade, add a fresh batch of the oil blend and

shake the bottle.

- These blends also make a great body or bath oil. Mix the oils with 2 oz. (1/4 cup) of your preferred carrier oil.

32. Fibromyalgia Buster Blend

Fibromyalgia sufferers deal with constant, chronic pain on a daily basis. This blend should help with the pain. It's for adult usage, to be applied topically, and can be diluted to suit.

Ingredients:

- 10 ml roller bottle
- 20 drops of Chamomile essential oil (e.g. Cape Chamomile)
- 20 drops of Lavender essential oil
- 20 drops of Wild Orange essential oil
- 20 drops of Marjoram essential oil
- fractionated Coconut oil

Directions:

- Pour the oils into the bottle first. Top off the bottle with the fractionated coconut oil.
- Close the bottle tightly, then shake to mix.
- Apply this blend to the bottom of your feet, abdomen, and inner wrists.

33. Insect Repellant

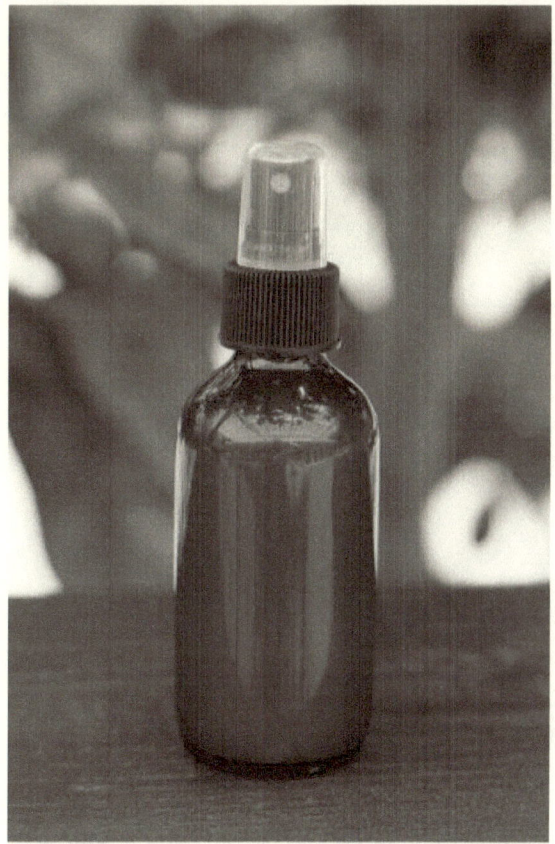

This bug spray should help you to rid your home of unwanted insects.

Ingredients:

- 2 oz. of distilled or boiled Water
- 1.5 oz. of Witch Hazel or Vodka
- 30 drops of Citronella essential oil
- 25 drops of Peppermint essential oil
- 15 drops of Tea Tree essential oil
- 1 tsp. of Jojoba oil (if used, add only 1 oz. of Vodka or Witch Hazel)

Directions:

Find a dark, clean 4 oz. spray bottle and fill it with water. Combine the witch hazel or vodka and about 50-75 total drops of essential oils with the water by shaking the bottle well. You can apply by spraying the blend directly on clothing or exposed skin. You can use every couple hours, or as needed. Avoid spraying into your eyes, mouth, or nose. Store away from direct sunlight or heat. This blend could also keep pests off the dog with a couple spritzes on the collar.

34. Perfume

Essential oils can also be used to create lovely smelling perfumes. Below is a simple recipe to get you started doing this. The blend is for adult usage.

Ingredients:

- 12-20 drops total of *Base tone essential oils* (choose from the list below):
  - Cedarwood
  - Vanilla
  - Vetiver
  - Ylang Ylang
  - Sandalwood
- 1 tsp. of homemade Vanilla extract (optional)
- 25-30 drops of *Middle tone essential oils*:
  - Rose
  - Lavender
  - Chamomile
  - Geranium
- 12-15 drops of *Top note essential oils*:
  - Bergamot
  - Wild Orange
  - Neroli
- 4 oz. of Alcohol to preserve and meld scents (e.g. non-GMO Spiced Rum)

Directions:

- Find an opaque bottle. After you blend the oils let it rest in the bottle for 24-48 hours so scents can meld.
- Add alcohol, close bottle tightly, and shake to blend. Store for at least 30 days in a dark, cool place. That isn't necessary, but it can allow the alcohol scent to fade while the oils' scents intensify.

35. Acne Treatment

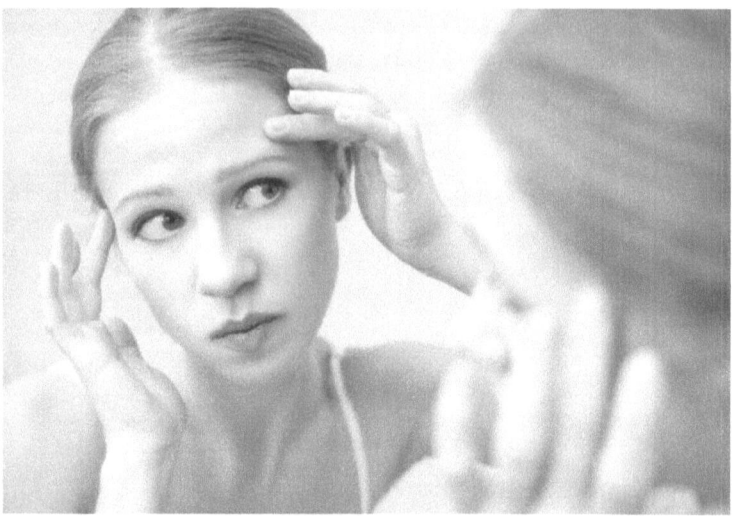

Clearing spotty skin and acne can be a nightmare. This blend is perfect for soothing these issues. They are for young adult (12+) to adult usage, to be applied topically, and can be diluted to suit.

Ingredients:

- 10 drops of Lavender essential oil
- 7 drops of Tea Tree essential oil
- 3 drops of Geranium essential oil
- 30 mL of Jojoba oil

Directions:

Find a dark, glass bottle. Add Jojoba oil and then the essential oils. Close the bottle and shake gently to blend; you will need to shake the bottle before each use. Treat the affected area by applying a small amount twice a day. Note: Avoid use on lips, nose, and eyes. Alternate ingredients: you can replace Tea Tree with Lemongrass. And, you can replace Jojoba oil with Aloe Vera gel.

36. Hair Serum

Stress, age, and even giving birth can thin your hair, make it brittle, or cause it to lose its luster. But this hair serum blend could help bring back some shine and thickness to your hair. So, here is a recipe for adult usage, which is to be applied topically. Refer to the "Dilution" chapter of this book if you wish to change it at all.

Ingredients:

- 2 oz. dark glass dropper bottle
- Almost 2 oz. of Castor oil
- 10 drops of Rosemary essential oil
- 5 drops of Lavender essential oil
- 5 drops of Ylang Ylang essential oil

Directions:

Find a dropper bottle, then pour in the Castor oil. Add the drops of essential oils, close dropper lid, and shake to mix the blend. Each morning, massage into your scalp. Wash your hair after waiting 20 minutes. If you aren't a morning person, this can also work if you apply the blend before going to bed. Note: Make this blend with 1 tsp. of witch hazel (to replace Castor oil) and about 2 oz. of distilled water to apply more frequently and feel less oily.

37. Calming Massage

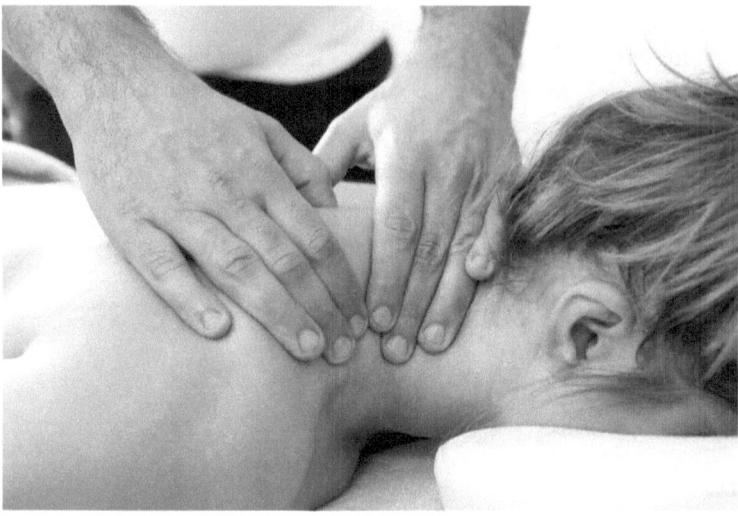

After a hectic and crazy day, there is nothing nicer than a calming massage. This blend is perfect for adult usage. It is to be applied topically and can be diluted to suit.

Ingredients:

- 6 drops of Anise essential oil
- 15 drops of Rose essential oil (5% in Jojoba)
- 6 drops of Nutmeg essential oil
- 60 mL of Carrier oil

Directions:

Find 1 oz. amber bottle. Add essential oils to carrier oil of your choice, then mix well. Massage into mid back, back of neck or upper chest. This blend can produce calm and relieve stress.

38. Congestion Recipe

Here is a brilliant blend for helping with nasal congestion. It is for adult use, to be taken topically or aromatically, and can be diluted to suit.

Ingredients:

- 10 drops of Eucalyptus Globulous essential oil
- 10 drops of Eucalyptus Radiata essential oil
- 10 drops of Rosemary essential oil
- 10 drops of Lavender essential oil
- 10 drops of Tea Tree essential oil
- 1 tbsp. of preferred Carrier oil

Directions:

Blend essential oils and carrier oil, then massage into back and upper chest. Or, you can inhale the blend by placing 3 drops of the oils into a tissue: inhale once, pause, then inhale again. These oils can help loosen congestion and fight bacterial and viral infections as they lift your spirit.

39. Homemade All Purpose Cleaner

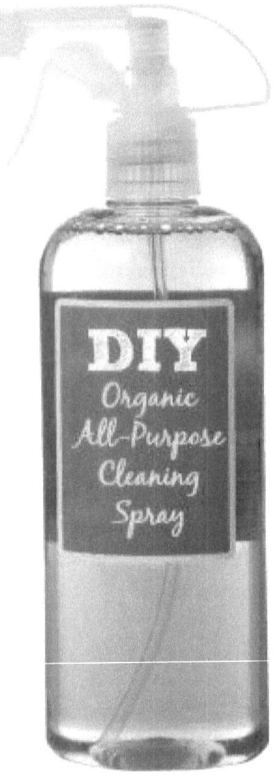

Here is a great recipe to help you clean your home.

Ingredients:

- 1 teaspoon of Borax
- 1/4 cup of White Vinegar
- 2 cups of Water
- 15 drops of Lemon essential oil
- 15 drops of Lavender essential oil

Directions:

Find a large, glass pitcher or measuring cup with a spout. Boil the water, then pour it into the cup or pitcher. Add borax and stir until it is completely dissolved, then add vinegar. Let this mixture cool. Once cool, pour into a spray bottle. Add drops of essential oils.

40. Letting Go Blend

This blend is perfect for working through anger and aggression. It has been developed for adult usage. Apply the blend topically and refer to the "Dilution" chapter of this book if necessary.

Ingredients:

- 3 drops of Cypress essential oil
- 4 drops of Ylang Ylang essential oil
- 2 drops of Frankincense essential oil
- 5 drops of Bergamot essential oil
- 7 drops of Geranium essential oil
- 4 drops of Patchouli essential oil
- 2 drops of Clary Sage essential oil

Directions:

Mix all oils together in a dark glass container. Place the blend on bottoms of feet, over liver and heart areas.

41. Increased Vitality Blend

Sometimes, just getting through a day is challenging enough! This recipe is perfect for increasing your vitality levels or motivation. It's for adult usage, to be applied topically and can be diluted to suit.

Ingredients:

- 5 drops of Black Pepper essential oil
- 5 drops of Lime essential oil
- 5 drops of Orange essential oil
- 5 drops of Frankincense essential oil
- 5-10 mL of Carrier oil (Almond, Grapeseed, fractionated Coconut oil)

Directions:

Mix essential oils in 5-10 mL roll-on bottle. Top off the bottle with Almond oil, Grapeseed, or fractionated Coconut oil. Roll on wrists 2 times a day.

42. Good Health

This immune system boosting blend is perfect for those under-the-weather days. It is for adult usage, to be applied topically, and can be diluted to suit.

Ingredients:

- 40 drops of Lavender essential oil
- 20 drops of Tea Tree essential oil
- 10 drops of Roman Chamomile essential oil
- 10 drops of Lemon essential oil

Directions:

Find an empty amber bottle. Blend oils, add to bottle, and fill remaining space with a carrier or massage oil of your choice. Apply just under your nose to immediately enjoy the blend's benefits. This relaxing blend will help you rest while your immune system fights the illness.

43. Beautiful Skin Recipes

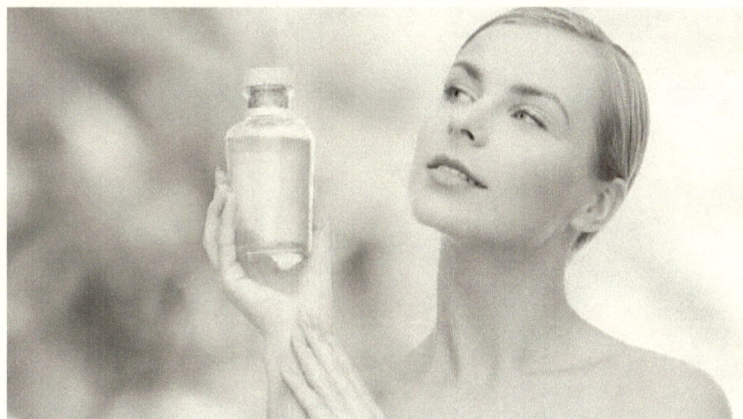

Nice-looking skin is something all people can benefit from! The two blends below are effective skin creams. They are for adult usage, to be applied topically, and can be diluted to suit.

Rejuvenating Facial Elixir Ingredients:

- 10 mL of Jojoba oil, Macadamia oil, or Olive Squalane
- 10 mL of Rosehip oil
- 4 drops of Frankincense essential oil
- 2 drops of Lavender essential oil
- 2 drops of Geranium essential oil

Antiaging Facial Serum Ingredients:

- 5 mL of Rosehip oil
- 5 mL of Macadamia oil
- 10 mL of Olive Squalane
- 4 drops of Frankincense essential oil
- 4 drops of Lavender essential oil

Directions:

Mix either of the blends above into a 20 mL pipette bottle. Massage a few drops into your skin; it will quickly absorb leaving you with a beautiful complexion. Both of these blends are suitable for all skin types and are to be applied to your face as part of your daily skin-care regimen.

44. Increased Metabolism

Increasing your metabolism can assist you in the fight against gaining weight, and this blend can help you in this mission. This recipe is for adult usage, to be used internally (with advice from an expert if you're a beginner in essential oil use), and can be diluted to suit.

Ingredients:

- 2 drops of Peppermint essential oil
- 2 drops of Grapefruit essential oil
- 2 drops of Lemon essential oil
- 12 drops of Coconut oil

Directions:

Consume by adding blend to a weight-loss capsule. Take one with a glass of water every day after your first meal.

45. Mood Enhancers

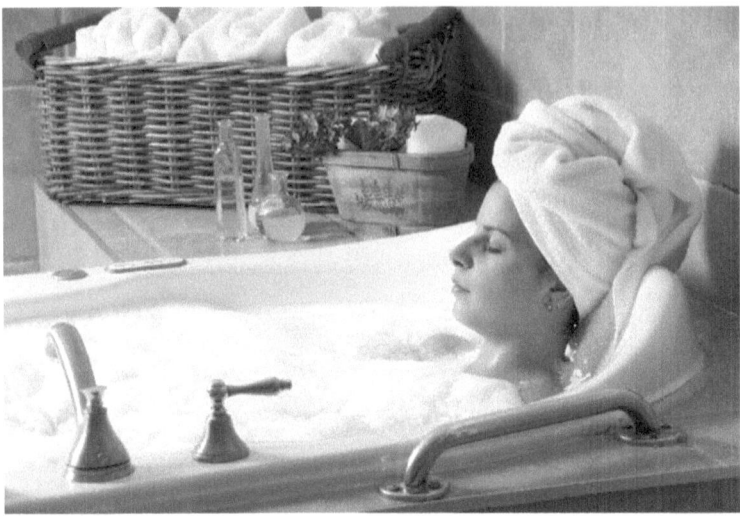

Having a nice, hot, soothing bath can instantly lift your mood anyway, but adding these essential oils will make it even better!

- *Blend to Combat Anger:*
  - o 3 drops of Orange essential oil
  - o 2 drops of Patchouli essential oil
- *Anxiety Blend:*
  - o 3 drops of Lavender essential oil
  - o 2 drops of Clary Sage essential oil
- *Blend to Help with Depression:*
  - o 3 drops of Bergamot essential oil
  - o 2 drops of Clary Sage essential oil
- *Energizing Blend:*
  - o 3 drops of Bergamot essential oil
  - o 2 drops of Rosemary essential oil
- *Blend to Ease Loneliness:*
  - o 2 drops of Bergamot essential oil
  - o 3 drops of Clary Sage essential oil
- *Stress Relieving Blend:*
  - o 3 drops of Clary Sage essential oil

- o   1 drop of Lemon essential oil
- o   1 drop of Lavender essential oil
- **Blends to Ease the Winter Blues:**
  - o   3 drops of Orange *and* 2 drops of Grapefruit essential oils
  - o   *or* 3 drops of Bergamot *and* 2 drops of Clary Sage essential oils
- **Blend to Ease Fear:**
  - o   3 drops of Grapefruit essential oil
  - o   2 drops of Bergamot essential oil
- **Blend to Help Increase Confidence**
  - o   3 drops of Orange essential oil
  - o   2 drops of Rosemary essential oil
- **Blends to Enhance Memory and Concentration:**
  - o   3 drops of Rosemary *and* 2 drops of Lemon essential oils
  - o   *or* 2 drops of Peppermint *and* 3 drops of Lemon essential oils

46. Ease Your Aches And Pains

For a relaxing way to ease your aches and pains, use this blend. It's for adult usage, to be used aromatically, and can be diluted to suit.

Ingredients:

- 2 drops of Lavender essential oil
- 1 drop of Chamomile essential oil
- 1 drop of Rose essential oil

Directions:

These oils are to be added to a hot bath to ease aches and pains.

47. Common Cold Blend

Below is a recipe to help you get over the nightmare that is the common cold. It has been designed for adult usage, to be used aromatically – in a bath or in a diffuser, and can be diluted to suit.

Ingredients:

- 2 drops of Lavender essential oil
- 2 drops of Rosemary essential oil
- 2 drops of Eucalyptus essential oil
- 2 tsp. of Milk or Cream

Directions:

Blend essential oils with milk or cream. Add to warm bath, stir, then soak. You could also apply this blend aromatically by placing in a diffuser without milk or cream.

48. Spice Up Your Love Life

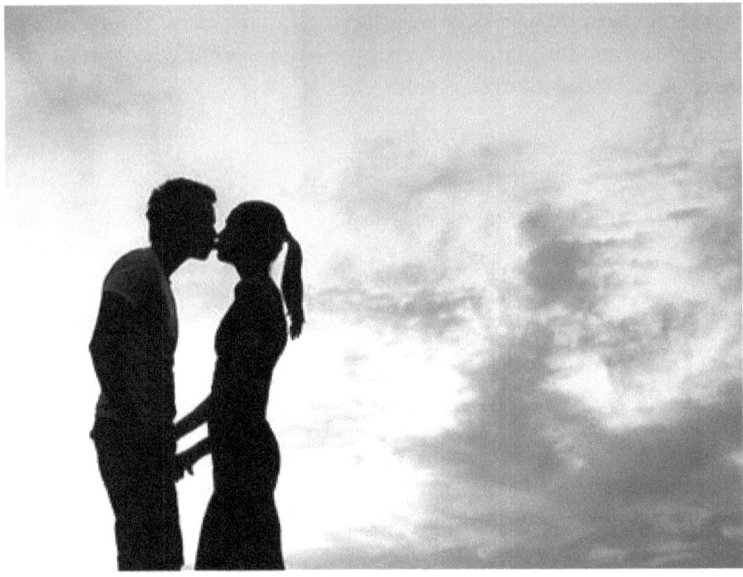

Even your love life can be helped by using essential oils, starting with this blend below. This is for adult usage and can be diluted to suit.

Ingredients:

- 2 drops of Sandalwood essential oil
- 3 drops of Ylang Ylang essential oil
- 1 drop of Patchouli essential oil or Rosemary essential oil

Directions:

Add the blend to your bath or diffuser to use aromatically.

49. Calming Massage Oil

Below is a very effective blend for calming down while facing everyday stresses. It is for adult usage, to be applied topically, and can be diluted to suit.

Ingredients:

- 6 drops of Petitgrain essential oil
- 5 drops of Orange essential oil
- 4 drops of Neroli essential oil
- 15 mL of preferred Carrier oil

Directions:

Blend essential oils with carrier oil, shake well. Massage into back and shoulders.

50. Flu Bomb

Getting rid of influenza can be a nightmare, which is why we have included this recipe. This is for adult usage, to be taken aromatically, and can be diluted to suit.

Ingredients:

- 15 drops of Thieves essential oil blend
- 15 drops of Tea Tree essential oil
- 15 drops of Lemon essential oil
- 10 drops of Oregano essential oil
- fractionated Coconut oil

Directions:

Find a glass roll-on bottle. Combine the essential oils, add to the bottle. Use the fractionated Coconut oil to fill remaining space. Apply every hour to the bottom of your feet or along your spine when you're sick; use as a preventative measure by applying twice a day. If you don't want to apply topically, add the mixture to capsules to consume orally when you're sick.

So, now you have seen how easy it is to create your own essential oil recipes at home. The ones used in this book will get you started, but there are plenty of online resources filled with more for you to try.

For example:

Aromaweb *at www.aromaweb.com/recipes*

Natural Living Ideas *at www.naturallivingideas.com/50-essential-oil-diffuser-recipes/*

Homemade Mommy *at www.homemademommy.net/recipes/diy-beauty-recipes-essential-oils-resources*

2 MOST COMMON MISTAKES FOR ESSENTIAL OIL USE

Below are the two most common mistakes in the use of essential oils, and suggestions on how to avoid them:

1.   *Essential oil overdose: Using too much, too often.*

If you're a regular user of essential oils, there is a good chance that you are also someone who prefers to put very little medication in your body. You understand that when you put a medication in your body, the medication needs to be detoxified through your liver or kidney systems. This detox process takes time and can be hard work for your liver and kidneys, many times causing toxicity side effects.

The same is true for essential oils. In no way do essential oils have the same side effects, but just like a medication, each person's constitution is different and will respond differently to essential oils and the amount you use. To avoid overusing essential oils, it is recommended **to approach essential oils thoughtfully and sparingly.**

2.   *Unbalanced use of essential oils.*

Some essential oils **are heating to the body and some are cooling**. For example, during the winter, a person should use less Peppermint essential oils (or other mint oils). Because mint oils are very cooling, they can do an excellent job to calm down the digestive system, but if overused during the winter, it can really mess up your digestion long term.

On the other hand, if a person uses something like Clove or Cinnamon oil, these are both warming. If you are someone who already has a warm constitution or has too much internal heat, using too many warming essential oils could cause hormonal, headache, blood pressure, or heart problems. Women, or even men, can develop hot flashes from using too many warming oils. These warming essential oils need time to properly clear through the liver. Unwanted symptoms from warming oils can especially pop up during the summer months.

The goal with essential oils is to use them in a balanced way by appropriately using cooling and warming oils together.

It's also advisable to refer to the "Safety" chapter of this book before using essential oils and to speak to a health professional if you have any questions.

GLOSSARY OF ESSENTIAL OIL TERMS

When dealing with essential oils, there are some terms that may be useful for you to know. Here is a glossary list.

Abortifacient	Capable of inducing abortion
Absolute	The most concentrated form of fragrance obtained when distilling a concrete
Adulterate	This is when unscrupulous companies mix pure essential oils with a base oil - thereby watering down the essential oil - but then still sell the 'watered down' oil as 100% pure essential oil. This is a huge problem in the essential oil market, as people are tempted to adulterate their oils for higher profit margins.
Acetylcholine	Is a fluid used in the transmission of information from one nerve ending to another
Allergy	Hypersensitivity caused by a foreign substance
Alopecia	Baldness – can be temporary or permanent
Alterative	Correcting disordered bodily functions
Amenorrhoea	The absence of menstruation
Anaerobic	Type of organism that does not require

	oxygen
Analgesic	Relieving or deadening pain
Anaphrodisiac	Lessening sexual desire
Anemia	Deficiency of either quantity or quality of red corpuscles in the blood
Anesthetic	Pain relieving by loss of sensation
Annual	Plant that completes its life cycle in one year
Anodyne	Stills pain and quieten disturbed feelings
Anosmic	Loss of smell
Anthelmintic	A vermifuge, destroying or expelling intestinal worms
Anti-acid	Combats acid in the body
Anti-arthritic	An agent which helps to combat arthritis
Anti-allergenic	Reduces symptoms of allergies
Antibacterial	Fights bacterial growth
Antibiotic	Fights infection in the body by preventing the growth or destroying bacteria
Anti-convulsant	Helps control convulsions
Anti-depressant	Helps to counteract depression and lifts the mood
Anti-dontalgic	Relieves toothache
Anti-emetic	Reduces the severity or incidence of vomiting
Anti-fungal	Prevents the growth of fungi
Anti-galactagogue	Impedes or lessens the flow of milk
Anti-hemorrhagic	A substance preventing or combating

	bleeding
Antihistamine	Counteracts allergic reaction
Anti-infectious	Prevents against infection
Anti-microbial	A substance reducing or resisting microbes
Antioxidant	A substance to prevent or delay oxidation
Anti-parasitic	Acts against parasites
Anti-phlogistic	Counteracts inflammation
Anti-pruritic	Relieves or prevents sensation of itching
Anti-pyretic	Reduces fever
Anti-rheumatic	An agent which helps to combat rheumatism
Anti-sclerotic	Helps to prevent hardening of arteries
Anti-seborrheic	Helps control the oily secretion from sweat glands
Antiseptic	A substance helping to control infection
Anti-spasmodic	A substance to help prevent and ease spasms and relieve cramps
Anti-sudorific	A substance to help lessen sweating
Anti-toxic	Antidote or treatment to counteract the effects of poison
Anti-tussive	Relieves coughing
Aperient	Mild laxative
Aphonia	Loss of voice
Aphrodisiac	Increasing sexual desire and sexual functioning
Apoplexy	Sudden loss of consciousness, a stroke or sudden hemorrhage

Aromatherapy	The therapeutic use of essential oils
Arrhythmia	Irregular or loss of heartbeat rhythm
Arteriosclerosis	Hardening of the arteries
Astringent	Causing contraction of organic tissue
Atherosclerosis	Accumulation of fatty deposits on the inside walls of arteries
Atony	Lack of muscle tone
Bactericidal	An agent destroying bacteria
Balsam	Water soluble, semi-solid or viscous resinous exudate similar to that of gum
Balsamic	Soothing medicine or application having the qualities of balsam
Bechic	Anything referring to coughing, or an agent relieving cough
Biennial	A plant completing its life cycle in two years, without flowering the first year
Bilious	A condition caused by an excessive secretion of bile
Blepharitis	Inflammation of the eyelids
Calmative	A sedative
Carcinogenic	A substance that promotes cancer or cancerous growths
Cardiac	Pertaining to the heart
Carminative	Settles the digestive system and relieves flatulence
Carrier oil	An oil which is used to dilute essential oils for the purpose of massage - see fixed oils
Cellulite	An "orange peel" effect caused by local

	accumulation of fat and waste products
Cephalic	A substance stimulating and clearing the mind
Chemotypes	The same botanical species occurring in other forms due to different growth conditions
Chi / Qi	Chinese term referring to the essential life force
Cholagogue	Stimulating the secretion of bile into the duodenum
Cholecystokenetic	Agent that stimulates the contraction of the gall bladder
Choleretic	Helps the liver to excrete bile, leading to greater bile flow
Cholesterol	Is a steroid alcohol found in red blood cells, bile, nervous tissue and animal fat
Cicatrisation	Formation of scar tissue
Cicatrisant	Agent promoting healing by scar tissue formation
Cirrhosis	Chronic inflammation and degeneration of any organ (normally in the liver)
Clinical trial	A controlled study to look at the effectiveness of a specific ingredient or application
Cohobation	Is a process in the extraction method of especially rose essential oil, to ensure a "complete" oil
Cold pressed	Refers to a method of extraction where no external heat is applied during the process
Colic	Pain due to contraction of the muscle of the abdominal organs
Colitis	Inflammation of the colon

Concrete	A waxy concentrate semi-solid essential oil extract, made from plant material, and is used to make an absolute
Constipation	A state where normal bowel functions are not present
Cutaneous	Pertaining to the skin
Cystitis	Bladder inflammation
Cytophylactic	Action of increasing the leukocyte activity to defend the body against infection
Cytotoxic	Toxic to all cells
Decoction	A herbal preparation made by boiling the material and reducing it to a concentration
Decongestant	A substance which helps to relieve congestion
Demulcent	An agent protecting mucus membranes and helps stop irritation
Depurative	Helps to detoxify and to combat impurities in the blood and body
Dermatitis	Inflammation of the skin
Detoxifier	Helps to detoxify and to combat impurities in the blood and body
Diaphoretic	A substance which helps to promote perspiration
Diffuser	A device which helps to release the fragrance molecules into the air
Distillation	A method of extraction used in the manufacture of essential oils
Diuretic	Helps to produce urine and remove water from the body
Dysmenorrhoea	Painful menstruation

Dysuria	Pain or difficulty in urinating
Edema	Water retention
Emetic	Inducing vomiting
Emmenagogue	Inducing or assisting menstruation
Emollient	Softening and soothing to the skin
Emphysema	Degenerative disease of the lungs where the air sacs become enlarged
Endocrine	Pertaining to the ductless glands
Engorgement	Congestion or fullness of the tissue
Enteritis	Inflammation of the mucus membranes of the intestine
Enuresis	Involuntary urinating
Enzyme	Protein produced by living cells which catalyze biochemical reactions
Erethism	Abnormal state of irritation or excitement
Essential oil	Volatile aromatic liquid constituting the odorous principles of botanical matter
Exocrine	Pertaining to a gland with a duct, secreting directly onto outside surface of organism
Expectorant	A substance that helps to expel mucus from the lungs
Expression	Is an extraction method where essential oils are pressed to obtain the oil
Exudates	Natural material secreted by plants - can be spontaneous or after damage to plant
Febrifuge	Helps to combat fever
Fibrillation	Rapid twitching of muscle fiber

Fixative	Material that slows evaporation of volatile components in perfume
Fixed oils	Vegetable oils obtained from plants that are fatty and non-volatile
Flower water	The water resulting from the distillation of essential oils, which still contains some of the properties of the plant material used in the extraction
Fold	Refers to the percentage of terpenes removed by re-distillation - single fold to five-fold
Fractionated oils	Refers to oils that have been re-distilled, either to have terpenes removed or to remove other substances
Fungicide	A substance which destroys fungal infections
Galactagogue	Helps to increase milk secretion
Gemicidal	An agent that destroys micro-organisms
Gingivitis	Inflammation of the gums
Glossitis	Inflammation of the tongue
Halitosis	Bad breath
Hematuria / Haematuria	Presence of blood in the urine
Hemorrhoids	Piles which are dilated rectal veins
Hemostatic	Helps to stop bleeding
Hepatic	Pertaining to the liver
Hepatoxic	An agent having a toxic or harmful effect on the liver
Herpes	Inflammation of the skin or mucus membranes

Hormone	A product from living cells that produces a specific activity of cells remote from its point of origin
Hybrid	A plant created by fertilization of one species by another
Hydrodiffusion	Is a distillation method of essential oil extraction where the steam is produced above the botanical material and then percolates down
Hydrosol	Floral water
Hyperglycemia / Hyperglycaemia	Excess of sugar in the blood
Hypertension	High blood pressure
Hypocholesterolemia	Lowering of the cholesterol content of the blood
Hypoglycemia	Lowered blood sugar levels
Hypotension	Abnormally low blood pressure
Hypoxia	A shortage of oxygen
In vitro	In a test tube
In vivo	In a living body
Infused oil	An oil produced by steeping the macerated botanical material in oil until the oil has taken on some of the material's properties
Infusion	Herbal remedy made by steeping the plant material in water
Laxative	A substance that helps with bowel movements
Leukocyte	White blood cells responsible for fighting disease
Leucocytosis	Raises number of white blood cells in the

	blood
Leucorrhoea	Whitish vaginal discharge
Lipolytic	Causing lipolysis which is the chemical disintegration of fats
Macerate	To soak until soft
Massage therapist	A person qualified to perform therapeutic massage on people
Massage therapy	The manipulation of soft tissue to enhance health and general well-being
Menopause	The normal cessation of menstruation
Menorrhagia	Excessive blood loss during menstruation
Metrorrhagia	Uterine bleeding outside the normal menstrual cycle
Microbe	Minute living organism such as pathogenic bacteria and viruses
Mucilage	Substance containing demulcent gelatinous constituents
Mucolytic	Breaking down mucus
Myelin	Fatty material enveloping the majority of nerve cells
Narcotic	Substance inducing sleep
Nephritis	Inflammation of the kidneys
Nervine	Substance that strengthens and tones the nerves and nervous system
Neuralgia	Stabbing pain along a nerve pathway
Neurasthenia	Nervous exhaustion
Neurotoxin	A substance having a toxic or harmful effect on the nervous system

Oedema	Water retention
Oleo gum resin	Odoriferous exudation from botanical material consisting of essential oil, gum and resin
Oleoresin	Natural resinous exudation from plants or aromatic liquid preparation extracted from botanical material
Olfaction	Sense of smell
Olfactory bulb	The center where the processing of smell is started and is then passed onto other areas of the brain
Oliguria	Low volume of urine
Ophthalmia	Inflammation of the eye
Ostitis	Inflammation of the ear
Oxidation	Related to the addition of oxygen to an organic molecule, or the removal of electrons or hydrogen from the molecule
Palpitations	Undue awareness of heartbeat, or rapid heartbeat or abnormal rhythm of the heart
Parturient	Assisting and helping childbirth
Pathogenic	An agent causing or producing disease
Peptic	Pertaining to gastric secretions as well as areas affected by them
Perennial	A plant living for more than two years
Pharmacology	Medical science pertaining to drugs
Pharmacopoeia	Official book of drugs
Pheromone	Chemical messenger used between people
Phytohormones	Plant substances mimicking the actions of human hormones

Phytotherapy	Treatment of disease with plant material, including herbal medicine
Polypus	Non-malignant type of growth
Pomade	Perfumed fat obtained during the enfleurage extraction method
Prophylactic	Preventative of disease or infection
Prostatitis	Inflammation of the prostate gland
Pruritis	Itching
Psoriasis	A chronic skin disease characterized by red patches and silver scaling
Psychosomatic	Pertaining to the mind and body
Pulmonary	Pertaining to the lungs
Pyelitis	Inflammation of the kidneys
Pyorrhea / Pyorrhoea	Discharge of puss from the gums
Pyrosis	Heartburn
Rectification	Process of re-distilling essential oils to rid them of certain constituents
Renal	Pertaining to the kidneys
Resin	Natural or prepared product - natural resins are exudations from trees, prepared resins are oleoresins from which the essential oil has been removed
Resinoids	Perfumed material extracted from natural resinous material by solvent extraction
Resolvent	An agent that helps disperse swelling, or that helps absorption of new growth
Rhizome	Underground stem that lasts for more than one season

Rubefacient	Substance causing redness and possible irritation to the skin
Sciatica	Pain down the back of the legs in the area serviced by the sciatic nerve
Sclerosis	Hardening of tissue due to inflammation
Scrofula	Tuberculosis of the lymphatic glands
Seborrhea	Increased secretion of sebum
Sialogogue	An agent stimulating the secretion of saliva
Soporific	A substance which helps to induce sleep
Spermatorrhoea	Involuntary emission of sperm without orgasm
Splenic	Pertaining to the spleen
Stomachic	A substance which helps with the digestion and helps to improve appetite
Stomatitis	Inflammation of the mucus membranes of the mouth
Styptic	An agent that stops external bleeding
Sudorific	An agent causing sweating
Synergy	Agents working together and in harmony to produce an effect greater than the sum of the two separate agents
Synthetic	Refers to anything not of organic source
Tachycardia	Abnormally increased heartbeat
Tannin	An astringent substance that helps seal tissues
Terpeneless	Essential oil from which monoterpene hydrocarbons have been removed
Thrombosis	The formation of a blood clot

Thrush	A fungal infection in the mouth or vaginal area
Tic	Repetitive twitching
Tincture	Referring to either a herbal or perfume material prepared in an alcohol base
Tracheitis	Inflammation of the windpipe
Tuber	Swollen part of underground stem of one year's duration and capable of new growth
Unguent	A soothing or healing salve or balm
Urticaria	Weal on the skin
Vasoconstrictor	An agent causing the contraction of blood vessel walls
Vasodilator	An agent causing the dilation of blood vessel walls
Vermifuge	An agent expelling intestinal worms
Volatile	Substance that is unstable and evaporates easily, like an essential oil
Vulnerary	An agent applied externally which helps to heal wounds and sores and helps to prevent tissue degeneration

RESOURCES

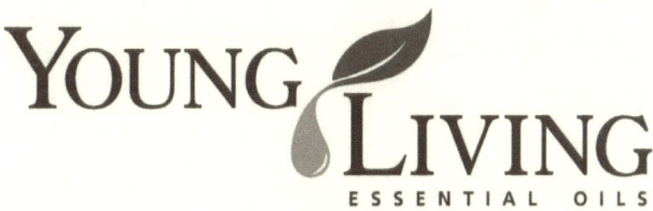

www.youngliving.com

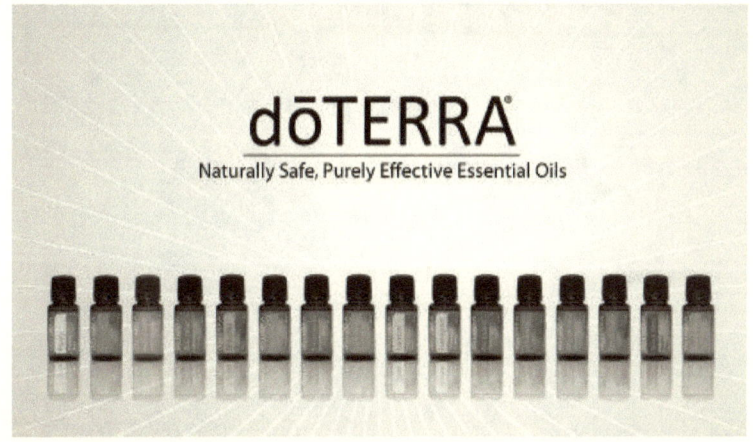

www.doterra.com

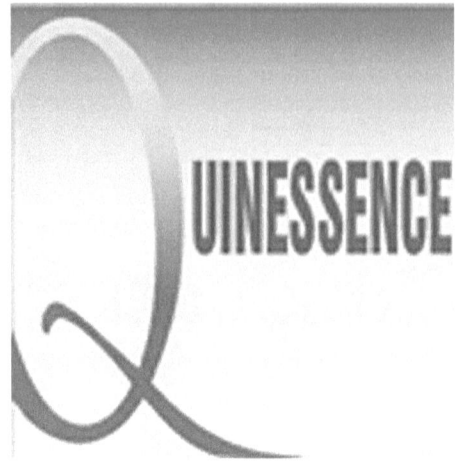

www.quinessence.com

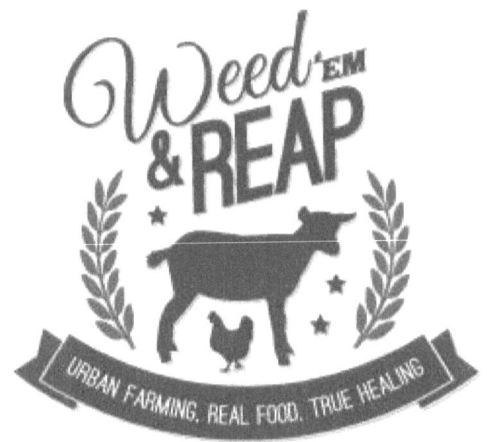

www.weedemandreap.com

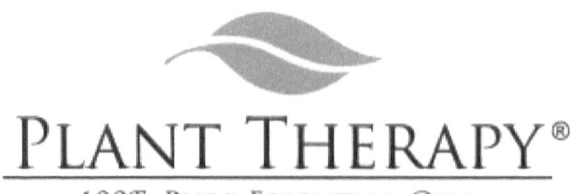

www.planttherapy.com

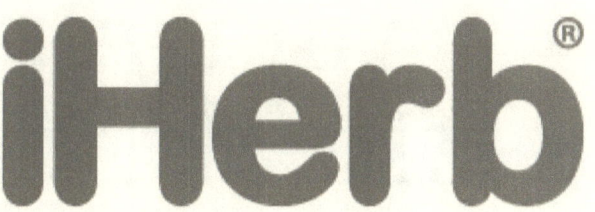

www.iherb.com

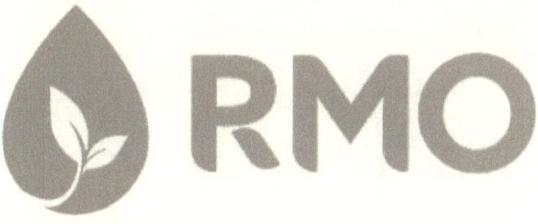

www.rockymountainoils.com

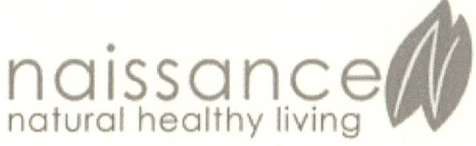

www.enaissance.co.uk

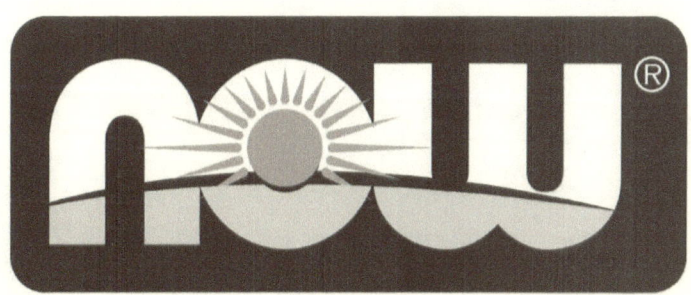

Nutrition for Optimal Wellness™

www.nowfoods.com

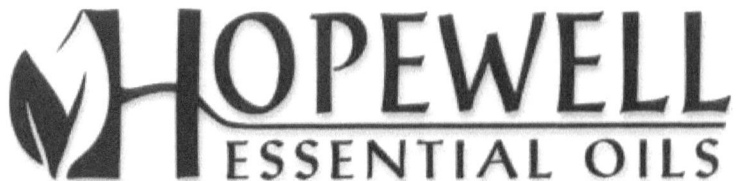

hopewelloils.com

www.naturallythinking.com

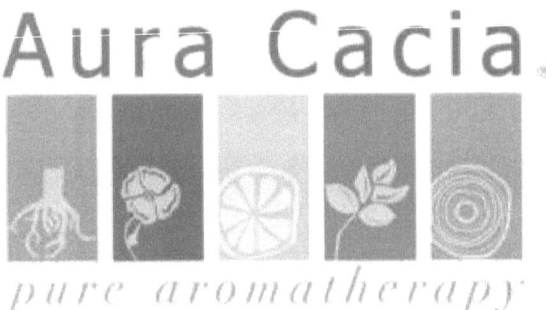

www.auracacia.com

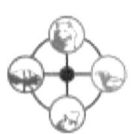
Native American Nutritionals

www.nativeamericannutritionals.com

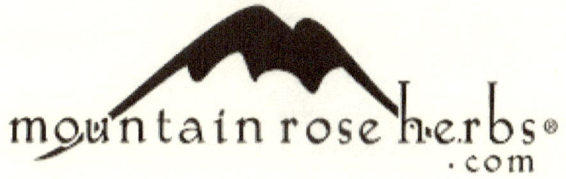

www.mountainroseherbs.com

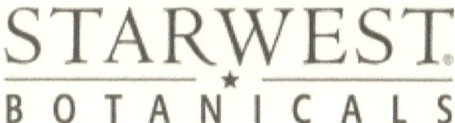

www.starwest-botanicals.com

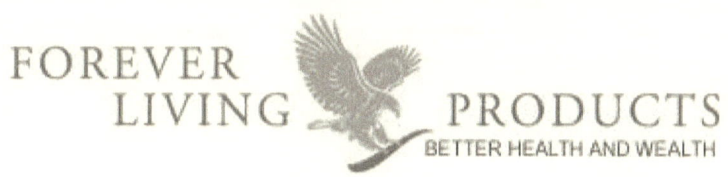

foreverliving.com

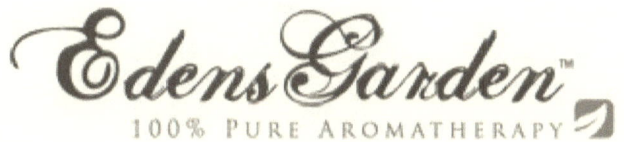

www.edensgarden.com

FAQ

1. Why is it close to impossible to find pure, therapeutic-grade essential oil?

This is because hundreds of pounds, at the very least, of materials are required to make just one pound of pure, therapeutic-grade oil. Consider Rose oil, it could take as much as 60 roses to produce just one drop! Unfortunately, companies often take short cuts to save money, so you will need to do your research to ensure you're getting what you want.

2. Where should you apply essential oils?

Essential oils can be applied almost anywhere on the skin – as long as you avoid your eye area. The "Application" chapter of this book goes into more detail on this subject.

3. What is the best way to administer essential oils?

As shown by the "Application" chapter of this book, essential oils can be taken aromatically, topically, internally, or externally. The best way to administer the oil is individual, to the ailment, the individual and the essential oil that you're using.

4. How do you use essential oils for weight loss?

There are many essential oils that can really help with weight loss – many regular oil users have a few that they recommend, such as in this guide from **Grass Fed Girl** *(www.grassfedgirl.com/6-essential-oils-for-weight-loss)*. Sandalwood, Grapefruit, Bergamot, Peppermint and Lemon are the most commonly recommended.

5. How can essential oils relieve stress?

More and more people are turning to essential oils to help manage stress in this fast-paced, highly stressed world we live in. Almost all essential oil users recommend Lavender as the most effective oil, but some sources also suggest Frankincense, Rose, Chamomile, and Vanilla.

6. Which essential oils should be avoided and why?

This is a very personalized matter – which is why you should always consult a health professional before using essential oils. This book gives you some general guidelines on this topic in the "Essential Oils to Avoid" chapter, and also the Safety information.

7. How much should I be paying for my essential oils?

Essential oils can cost anything from a couple of dollars to 50+ dollars. This price isn't *necessarily* a guide to how good the product is. You are much more likely to get a better picture of this by researching the company's reputation.

8. Can I ingest essential oils?

It is inadvisable to ingest essential oils – particularly if you are a beginner. If you *do* intend to do this, it is best to speak to a certified aromatherapist beforehand.

9. What are the best brands of essential oils?

The "Brands" chapter of this book covers the most popular. The most commonly known are doTerra and Young Living.

10. What are the best smelling essential oils?

Of course, this is a subject in which everyone will have a different opinion, but the most popular essential oils used for perfume are Jasmine Absolute, Bergamot, Lemon, Vetiver, Ylang Ylang, Cinnamon, Cedarwood, Vanilla, and Rose Otto essential oils. In fact, approximately 98% of the essential oils produced today are for the perfume industry. One of the most expensive perfumes in the world, "Joy Perfume by Jean Patou," contains Jasmine Absolute and Rose Otto essential oils. *Joy* essential oil blend from Young Living contains these oils, has no alcohol, and has a ton of benefits.

11. Where are the best places to buy essential oils online?

The "Brands" chapter of this book gives you the top essential oils and where to find their online stores.

12. Do essential oils have an expiry date?

Yes, essential oils will have expiration dates to keep users safe. **Aromaweb** (www.aromaweb.com/articles/essentialoilshelflife.asp) has an in-depth guide about this subject. It suggests that, as a broad rule of thumb, most essential oils are good for one year after the date of purchase, while some oils are claimed to have a lifespan of up to 10 years. In fact, if blended, essential oils will only be good while the carrier oil used is within its expiration date.

13. How should I use Rosemary essential oil?

Rosemary essential oil has 4 primary uses: contributes to hair growth, improves memory, liver detox and lowers cortisol. Visit website draxe.com/rosemary-oil-uses-benefits for more details of how you should use this oil for different ailments.

14. How should I use pure essential oils?

Use the "Pure vs. Quality" chapter of this book to find out more about pure essential oils. These oils must always be diluted using carrier oils to ensure that they are safe for use. This book has all the information you'll need to get the dilution ratio correct.

15. How do I know if the oils I'm ordering are 100% pure and not diluted by carrier oil?

Essential oils are generally sold pure, so users can dilute them to suit their needs. If this is ever different, it will be labelled very clearly.

16. What essential oils promote hair growth?

Aside from Rosemary, Ananda Apothecary has a long list of essential oils for hair care and growth. These include Clove, Cedarwood, Thyme, Lavender, and Ylang Ylang.

17. What's the difference between essence and essential oils?

A plant's essence is comprised of the vibrational energy, whereas essential oils represent and transfer the physical properties of a plant to a person to improve health and well-being.

18. What is the difference between essential oils and aromatherapy?

Aromatherapy is a scientific or medicinal therapy that employs natural extractions from plants to enhance health and well-being. **Essential oils** are those natural extractions. Both are used, separately or together, to help improve your physical and emotional well-being.

19. Which essential oils are safe to use if you are pregnant?

The "Pregnancy" section in this book goes into more detail on this subject. It is suggested that the essential oils that appear to be safe to use during pregnancy include:

- Cardamom
- Frankincense
- Geranium
- Neroli
- Patchouli
- Petitgrain
- Rosewood
- Rose
- Sandalwood
- And other nontoxic essential oils.

20. Are there any clinical studies to prove the healing properties of essential oils?

As essential oils rise in popularity, the number of studies being done increases. Most of the data from this can be found at the **NCBI** website at www.ncbi.nlm.nih.gov/pubmedhealth/PMH0032645.

CONCLUSION

So, as you can see from all of the information in this book, essential oils are one of the *best* ways to fight common ailments. They are **nontoxic, easy to use,** and **easy to make** – as shown by the "Recipes" chapter.

Not only that, the oils are a much more natural solution to your problems, which of course means that they have fewer side effects – and as anyone who has spent an extended period using traditional medicine will know, the side effects can sometimes be worse than the initial problem! Best of all, there is an essential oil treatment out there for absolutely anything, so there's really no reason to not at least give them a *try*.

WIDE ARRAY	of vital actions in body
SIGNIFICANT RANGE	of potencies
HELPS WITH	all major organs & systems
SAFE	with virtually no side effects
PROVEN	by thousands of studies
USED BY DOCTORS	and experts across the globe

One thought that may help mitigate the cost you incur by investing in essential oils is knowing they have a shelf life (noting a few exceptions) of **at least 5 years**. This is because they are *so* concentrated that a tiny amount is required for any use you have for them. Citrus oils are the only exception, you can see a reduction in strength after just a couple years.

This book has given you **everything that you need to get started** using essential oils - a Buying Guide, a selection of Top Oils to try, and a list of Resources to allow you to do your very own research in the areas that you are most interested in, whilst speaking to other essential oil users along the way.

Of course, it is always recommended to speak to a health professional before using any oils to confirm that they will suit you and to get advice on the best ways to take any particular oils.

ABOUT THE AUTHOR

Mary Jones became interested in herbal remedies early on in her life. She came to essential oils after years of looking for solutions to her problems in the medical world. Issues like allergies, weight loss, and lack of energy didn't really seem to have good solutions in traditional medicine. There were expensive treatments to be had, but often they did not work in the long term and were not as holistic as Mary wanted the treatments to be.

In her search for a solution, she came upon essential oils and aromatherapy. As she had learned about the stress-relieving power of aromatherapy, she began intensely studying essential oils – how they work, how they are used, how they are made, which are safe to use, and beyond. She travelled to study with those who had long used essential oils and taught others about their many uses. For decades, she has developed her knowledge about this subject.

One of Mary's life goals is to make the world a better, happier place, and her writings are definitely a testament to that. She did not want to keep all of her research and discoveries to herself. She has elected to share them, in a format that makes them available to just about everyone.

Now, after years of compiling information about the most beneficial and useful essential oils, Mary has written several books to introduce others to the knowledge she has gathered.

www.ingramcontent.com/pod-product-compliance
Lightning Source LLC
Chambersburg PA
CBHW030424290526

45786CB00001B/126